Nutrition Diagnosis:

A Critical Step in the Nutrition Care Process

American
Dietetic
Association

Nutrition Diagnosis: A Critical Step in the Nutrition Care Process

ISBN: 0-88091-358-4

10 9 8 7 6 5 4 3 2 1

Nutrition Diagnosis: A Critical Step in the Nutrition Care Process

Table of Contents

Please check the ADA Web site for additional materials

http://www.eatright.org. Sign in as a member and select Research from sidebar.
http://www.eatright.org. Sign in as a member and select Quality Management and Outcomes from the sidebar.

Nutrition Care Process and Model: ADA adopts road map to quality care and outcomes management

KAREN LACEY, MS, RD; ELLEN PRITCHETT, RD

The establishment and implementation of a standardized Nutrition Care Process (NCP) and Model were identified as priority actions for the profession for meeting goals of the ADA Strategic Plan to "Increase demand and utilization of services provided by members" and "Empower members to compete successfully in a rapidly changing environment" (1). Providing high-quality nutrition care means doing the right thing at the right time, in the right way, for the right person, and achieving the best possible results. Quality improvement literature shows that, when a standardized process is implemented, less variation and more predictability in terms of outcomes occur (2). When providers of care, no matter their location, use a process consistently, comparable outcomes data can be generated to demonstrate value. A standardized Nutrition Care Process effectively promotes the dietetics professional as the unique provider of nutrition care when it is consistently used as a systematic method to think critically and make decisions to provide safe and effective nutrition care (3).

This article describes the four steps of ADA's Nutrition Care Process and the overarching framework of the Nutrition Care Model that illustrates the context within which the Nutrition Care Process occurs. In addition, this article provides the rationale for a standardized process by which nutrition care is provided, distinguishes between the Nutrition Care Process and Medical Nutrition Therapy (MNT), and discusses future implications for the profession.

BACKGROUND

Prior to the adoption of this standardized Nutrition Care Process, a variety of nutrition care processes were utilized by practitioners and taught by dietetics educators. Other allied health professionals, including nursing, physical therapy, and occupational therapy, utilize defined care processes specific to their profession (4-6). When asked whether ADA should develop a standardized Nutrition Care Process, dietetics professionals were overwhelmingly in favor and strongly supportive of having a standardized Nutrition Care Process for use by registered dietitians (RD) and dietetics technicians, registered (DTR).

The Quality Management Committee of the House of Delegates (HOD) appointed a Nutrition Care Model Workgroup in May 2002 to develop a nutrition care process and model. The first draft was presented to the HOD for member input and review in September 2002. Further discussion occurred during the October 2002 HOD meeting, in Philadelphia. Revisions were made accordingly, and the HOD unanimously adopted the final version of the Nutrition Care Process and Model on March 31, 2003 "for implementation and dissemination to the dietetics profession and the Association for the enhancement of the practice of dietetics."

SETTING THE STAGE

Definition of Quality/Rationale for a Standardized Process

The National Academy of Science's (NAS) Institute of Medicine (IOM) has defined quality as "The degree to which health services for individuals and populations increase the likelihood of desired health outcomes and are consistent with current professional knowledge" (7,8). The quality performance of providers can be assessed by measuring the following: (a) their patients' outcomes (end-results) or (b) the degree to which providers adhere to an accepted care process (7,8). The Committee on Quality of Health Care in America further states that it is not acceptable to have a wide quality chasm, or a gap, between *actual* and *best possible* performance (9). In an effort to ensure that dietetics professionals can meet both requirements for quality performance noted above, the American Dietetic Association (ADA) supports a standardized Nutrition Care Process for the profession.

Standardized Process versus Standardized Care

ADA's Nutrition Care Process is a standardized process for dietetics professionals and not a means to provide standardized care. A standardized process refers to a consistent structure and framework used to provide nutrition care, whereas stan-

K. Lacey is lecturer and Director of Dietetic Programs at the University of Wisconsin-Green Bay, Green Bay. She is also the Chair of the Quality Management Committee. E. Pritchett is Director, Quality and Outcomes at ADA headquarters in Chicago, IL.

If you have questions regarding the Nutrition Care Process and Model, please contact Ellen Pritchett, RD, CPHQ, Director of Quality and Outcomes at ADA, epritchett@eatright.org

0002-8223/03/10308-0014$35.00/0
doi: 10.1053/jada.2003.50564

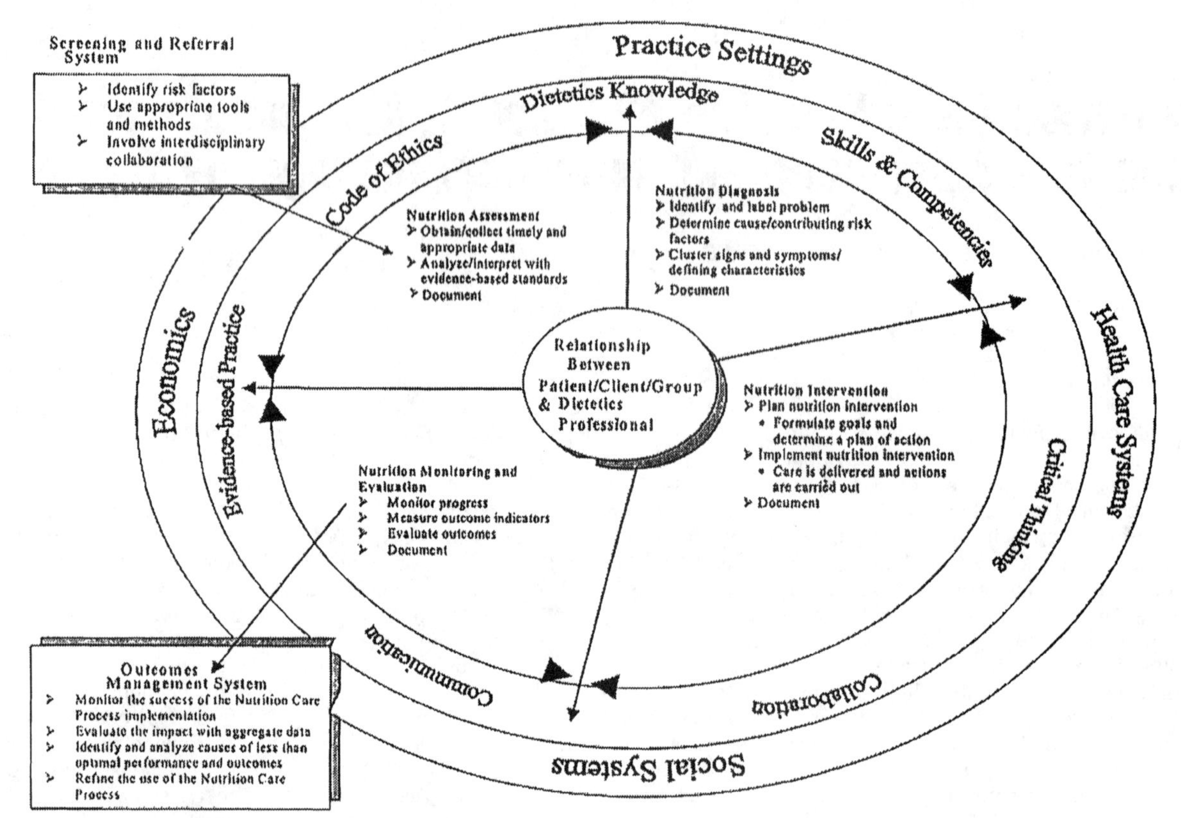

FIG 1. ADA Nutrition Care Process and Model.

dardized care infers that all patients/clients receive the same care. This process supports and promotes individualized care, not standardized care. As represented in the model (Figure 1), the relationship between the patient/client/group and dietetics professional is at the core of the nutrition care process. Therefore, nutrition care provided by qualified dietetics professionals should always reflect both the state of the science and the state of the art of dietetics practice to meet the individualized needs of each patient/client/group (10).

Using the NCP

Even though ADA's Nutrition Care Process will primarily be used to provide nutrition care to individuals in health care settings (inpatient, ambulatory, and extended care), the process also has applicability in a wide variety of community settings. It will be used by dietetics professionals to provide nutrition care to both individuals and groups in community-based agencies and programs for the purpose of health promotion and disease prevention (11,12).

Key Terms

To lay the groundwork and facilitate a clear definition of ADA's Nutrition Care Process, key terms were developed. These definitions provide a frame of reference for the specific components and their functions.

(a) Process is a series of connected steps or actions to achieve an outcome and/or any activity or set of activities that transforms inputs to outputs.

(b) Process Approach is the systematic identification and management of activities and the interactions between activities. A process approach emphasizes the importance of the following:

- understanding and meeting requirements;
- determining if the process adds value;
- determining process performance and effectiveness; and
- using objective measurement for continual improvement of the process (13).

(c) Critical Thinking integrates facts, informed opinions, active listening and observations. It is also a reasoning process in which ideas are produced and evaluated. The Commission on Accreditation of Dietetics Education (CADE) defines critical thinking as "transcending the boundaries of formal education to explore a problem and form a hypothesis and a defensible conclusion" (14). The use of critical thinking provides a unique strength that dietetics professionals bring to the Nutrition Care Process. Further characteristics of critical thinking include the ability to do the following:

- conceptualize;
- think rationally;
- think creatively;
- be inquiring; and
- think autonomously.

(d) Decision Making is a critical process for choosing the best action to meet a desired goal.

(e) Problem Solving is the process of the following:

- problem identification;
- solution formation;
- implementation; and
- evaluation of the results.

(f) Collaboration is a process by which several individuals or groups with shared concerns are united to address an identified problem or need, leading to the accomplishment of what each could not do separately (15).

DEFINITION OF ADA'S NCP

Using the terms and concepts described above, ADA's Nutrition Care Process is defined as "a systematic problem-solving method that dietetics professionals use to critically think and make decisions to address nutrition related problems and provide safe and effective quality nutrition care."

The Nutrition Care Process consists of four distinct, but interrelated and connected steps: (a) Nutrition Assessment, (b) Nutrition Diagnosis, (c) Nutrition Intervention, and d) Nutrition Monitoring and Evaluation. These four steps were finalized based on extensive review and evaluation of previous works describing nutrition care (16-24). Even though each step builds on the previous one, the process is not linear. Critical thinking and problem solving will frequently require that dietetics professionals revisit previous steps to reassess, add, or revise nutrition diagnoses; modify intervention strategies; and/or evaluate additional outcomes. Figure 2 describes each of these four steps in a similar format consisting of the following:

- definition and purpose;
- key components or substeps with examples as appropriate;
- critical thinking characteristics;
- documentation elements; and
- considerations for continuation, discontinuation, or discharge of care.

Providing nutrition care using ADA's Nutrition Care Process begins when a patient/client/group has been identified at nutrition risk and needs further assistance to achieve or maintain nutrition and health goals. It is also important to recognize that patients/clients who enter the health care system are more likely to have nutrition problems and therefore benefit from receiving nutrition care in this manner. The Nutrition Care Process cycles through the steps of assessment, diagnosis, intervention, and monitoring and evaluation. Nutrition care can involve one or more cycles and ends, ideally, when nutrition goals have been achieved. However, the patient/client/group may choose to end care earlier based on personal or external factors. Using professional judgment, the dietetics professional may discharge the patient/client/group when it is determined that no further progress is likely.

PURPOSE OF NCP

ADA's Nutrition Care Process, as described in Figure 2, gives dietetics professionals a consistent and systematic structure and method by which to think critically and make decisions. It also assists dietetics professionals to scientifically and holistically manage nutrition care, thus helping patients better meet their health and nutrition goals. As dietetics professionals consistently use the Nutrition Care Process, one should expect a higher probability of producing good outcomes. The Nutrition Care Process then begins to establish a link between quality and professional autonomy. Professional autonomy results from being recognized for what we do *well*, not just for who we are. When quality can be demonstrated, as defined previously by the IOM (7,8), then dietetics professionals will stand out as the preferred providers of nutrition services. The Nutrition Care Process, when used consistently, also challenges dietetics professionals to move beyond experience-based practice to reach a higher level of evidence-based practice (9,10).

The Nutrition Care Process does not restrict practice but acknowledges the common dimensions of practice by the following:

- defining a common language that allows nutrition practice to be more measurable;
- creating a format that enables the process to generate quantitative and qualitative data that can then be analyzed and interpreted; and
- serving as the structure to validate nutrition care and showing how the nutrition care that was provided does what it intends to do.

DISTINCTION BETWEEN MNT AND THE NCP

Medical Nutrition Therapy (MNT) was first defined by ADA in the mid-1990s to promote the benefits of managing or treating a disease with nutrition. Its components included an assessment of nutritional status of patients and the provision of either diet modification, counseling, or specialized nutrition therapies. MNT soon became a widely used term to describe a wide variety of nutrition care services provided by dietetics professionals. Since MNT was first introduced, dietetics professionals have gained much credibility among legislators and other health care providers. More recently, MNT has been redefined as part of the 2001 Medicare MNT benefit legislation to be "nutritional diagnostic, therapy, and counseling services for the purpose of disease management, which are furnished by a registered dietitian or nutrition professional" (25).

The intent of the NCP is to describe accurately the spectrum of nutrition care that can be provided by dietetics professionals. Dietetics professionals are uniquely qualified by virtue of academic and supervised practice training and appropriate certification and/or licensure to provide a comprehensive array of professional services relating to the prevention or treatment of nutrition-related illness (14,26). MNT is but one specific type of nutrition care. The NCP articulates the consistent and specific steps a dietetics professional would use when delivering MNT, but it will also be used to guide nutrition education and other preventative nutrition care services. One of the key distinguishing characteristics between MNT and the other nutrition services using the NCP is that MNT always involves an in-depth, comprehensive assessment and individualized care. For example, one individual could receive MNT for diabetes and also nutrition education services or participate in a community-based weight loss program (27). Each service would use the Nutrition Care Process, but the process would be implemented differently; the components of each step of the process would be tailored to the type of service.

By articulating the steps of the Nutrition Care Process, the commonalities (the consistent, standardized, four-step process) of nutrition care are emphasized even though the process is implemented differently for different nutrition services. With a standardized Nutrition Care Process in place, MNT should not be used to describe all of the nutrition services that dietetics professionals provide. As noted above, MNT is the only application of the Nutrition Care Process (28-31). This change in

	STEP 1. NUTRITION ASSESSMENT
Basic Definition & Purpose	**"Nutrition Assessment"** is the first step of the Nutrition Care Process. Its purpose is to obtain adequate information in order to identify nutrition-related problems. It is initiated by referral and/or screening of individuals or groups for nutritional risk factors. Nutrition assessment is a systematic process of obtaining, verifying, and interpreting data in order to make decisions about the nature and cause of nutrition-related problems. The specific types of data gathered in the assessment will vary depending on a) practice settings, b) individual/groups' present health status, c) how data are related to outcomes to be measured, d) recommended practices such as ADA's Evidence Based Guides for Practice and e) whether it is an initial assessment or a reassessment. Nutrition assessment requires making comparisons between the information obtained and reliable standards (ideal goals). Nutrition assessment is an on-going, dynamic process that involves not only initial data collection, but also continual reassessment and analysis of patient/client/group needs. Assessment provides the foundation for the nutrition diagnosis at the next step of the Nutrition Care Process.
Data Sources/Tools for Assessment	■ Referral information and/or interdisciplinary records ■ Patient/client interview (across the lifespan) ■ Community-based surveys and focus groups ■ Statistical reports; administrative data ■ Epidemiological studies
Types of Data Collected	■ Nutritional Adequacy (dietary history/detailed nutrient intake) ■ Health Status (anthropometric and biochemical measurements, physical & clinical conditions, physiological and disease status) ■ Functional and Behavioral Status (social and cognitive function, psychological and emotional factors, quality-of-life measures, change readiness)
Nutrition Assessment Components	■ Review dietary intake for factors that affect health conditions and nutrition risk ■ Evaluate health and disease condition for nutrition-related consequences ■ Evaluate psychosocial, functional, and behavioral factors related to food access, selection, preparation, physical activity, and understanding of health condition ■ Evaluate patient/client/group's knowledge, readiness to learn, and potential for changing behaviors ■ Identify standards by which data will be compared ■ Identify possible problem areas for making nutrition diagnoses
Critical Thinking	The following types of critical thinking skills are especially needed in the assessment step: ■ Observing for nonverbal and verbal cues that can guide and prompt effective interviewing methods; ■ Determining appropriate data to collect; ■ Selecting assessment tools and procedures (matching the assessment method to the situation); ■ Applying assessment tools in valid and reliable ways; ■ Distinguishing relevant from irrelevant data; ■ Distinguishing important from unimportant data; ■ Validating the data; ■ Organizing & categorizing the data in a meaningful framework that relates to nutrition problems; and ■ Determining when a problem requires consultation with or referral to another provider.
Documentation of Assessment	Documentation is an on-going process that supports all of the steps in the Nutrition Care Process. Quality documentation of the assessment step should be relevant, accurate, and timely. Inclusion of the following information would further describe quality assessment documentation: ■ Date and time of assessment; ■ Pertinent data collected and comparison with standards; ■ Patient/client/groups' perceptions, values, and motivation related to presenting problems; ■ Changes in patient/client/group's level of understanding, food-related behaviors, and other clinical outcomes for appropriate follow-up; and ■ Reason for discharge/discontinuation if appropriate.
Determination for Continuation of Care	If upon the completion of an initial or reassessment it is determined that the problem cannot be modified by further nutrition care, discharge or discontinuation from this episode of nutrition care may be appropriate.

FIG 2. ADA Nutrition Care Process.

STEP 2. NUTRITION DIAGNOSIS

Basic Definition & Purpose	**"Nutrition Diagnosis"** is the second step of the Nutrition Care Process, and is the identification and labeling that describes an actual occurrence, risk of, or potential for developing a nutritional problem that dietetics professionals are responsible for treating independently. At the end of the assessment step, data are clustered, analyzed, and synthesized. This will reveal a nutrition diagnostic category from which to formulate a specific nutrition diagnostic statement. Nutrition diagnosis should not be confused with medical diagnosis, which can be defined as a disease or pathology of specific organs or body systems that can be treated or prevented. A nutrition diagnosis changes as the patient/client/group's response changes. A medical diagnosis does not change as long as the disease or condition exists. A patient/client/group may have the medical diagnosis of "Type 2 diabetes mellitus"; however, after performing a nutrition assessment, dietetics professionals may diagnose, for example, "undesirable overweight status" or "excessive carbohydrate intake." Analyzing assessment data and naming the nutrition diagnosis(es) provide a link to setting realistic and measurable expected outcomes, selecting appropriate interventions, and tracking progress in attaining those expected outcomes.
Data Sources/Tools for Diagnosis	■ Organized and clustered assessment data ■ List(s) of nutrition diagnostic categories and nutrition diagnostic labels ■ Currently the profession does not have a standardized list of nutrition diagnoses. However ADA has appointed a Standardized Language Work Group to begin development of standardized language for nutrition diagnoses and intervention. (June 2003)
Nutrition Diagnosis Components (3 distinct parts)	**1. Problem (Diagnostic Label)** The nutrition diagnostic statement describes alterations in the patient/client/group's nutritional status. A diagnostic label (qualifier) is an adjective that describes/qualifies the human response such as: ■ Altered, impaired, ineffective, increased/decreased, risk of, acute or chronic. **2. Etiology (Cause/Contributing Risk Factors)** The related factors (etiologies) are those factors contributing to the existence of, or maintenance of pathophysiological, psychosocial, situational, developmental, cultural, and/or environmental problems. ■ Linked to the problem diagnostic label by words "related to" (RT) ■ It is important not only to state the problem, but to also identify the cause of the problem. □ This helps determine whether or not nutritional intervention will improve the condition or correct the problem. □ It will also identify who is responsible for addressing the problem. Nutrition problems are either caused directly by inadequate intake (primary) or as a result of other medical, genetic, or environmental factors (secondary). □ It is also possible that a nutrition problem can be the cause of another problem. For example, excessive caloric intake may result in unintended weight gain. Understanding the cascade of events helps to determine how to prioritize the interventions. □ It is desirable to target interventions at correcting the cause of the problem whenever possible; however, in some cases treating the signs and symptoms (consequences) of the problem may also be justified. ■ The ranking of nutrition diagnoses permits dietetics professionals to arrange the problems in order of their importance and urgency for the patient/client/group. **3. Signs/Symptoms (Defining Characteristics)** The defining characteristics are a cluster of subjective and objective signs and symptoms established for each nutrition diagnostic category. The defining characteristics, gathered during the assessment phase, provide evidence that a nutrition related problem exists and that the problem identified belongs in the selected diagnostic category. They also quantify the problem and describe its severity: ■ Linked to etiology by words "as evidenced by" (AEB); ■ The symptoms (subjective data) are changes that the patient/client/group feels and expresses verbally to dietetics professionals; and ■ The signs (objective data) are observable changes in the patient/client/group's health status.
Nutrition Diagnostic Statement (PES)	Whenever possible, a nutrition diagnostic statement is written in a PES format that states the Problem (P), the Etiology (E), and the Signs & Symptoms (S). However, if the problem is either a risk (potential) or wellness problem, the nutrition diagnostic statement may have only two elements, Problem (P), and the Etiology (E), since Signs & Symptoms (S) will not yet be exhibited in the patient. A well-written Nutrition Diagnostic Statement should be: 1. Clear and concise 2. Specific: patient/client/group-centered 3. Related to one client problem 4. Accurate: relate to one etiology 5. Based on reliable and accurate assessment data **Examples of Nutrition Diagnosis Statements (PES or PE)** ■ Excessive caloric intake (problem) "related to" frequent consumption of large portions of high fat meals (etiology) "as evidenced by" average daily intake of calories exceeding recommended amount by 500 kcal and 12-pound weight gain during the past 18 months (signs)

FIG 2 cont'd.

	■ Inappropriate infant feeding practice RT lack of knowledge AEB infant receiving bedtime juice in a bottle ■ Unintended weight loss RT inadequate provision of energy by enteral products AEB 6-pound weight loss over past month ■ Risk of weight gain RT a recent decrease in daily physical activity following sports injury
Critical Thinking	The following types of critical thinking skills are especially needed in the diagnosis step: ■ Finding patterns and relationships among the data and possible causes; ■ Making inferences ("if this continues to occur, then this is likely to happen"); ■ Stating the problem clearly and singularly; ■ Suspending judgment (be objective and factual); ■ Making interdisciplinary connections; ■ Ruling in/ruling out specific diagnoses; and ■ Prioritizing the relative importance of problems for patient/client/group safety.
Documentation of Diagnosis	Documentation is an on-going process that supports all of the steps in the Nutrition Care Process. Quality documentation of the diagnosis step should be relevant, accurate, and timely. A nutrition diagnosis is the impression of dietetics professionals at a given point in time. Therefore, as more assessment data become available, the documentation of the diagnosis may need to be revised and updated. Inclusion of the following information would further describe quality documentation of this step: ■ Date and time; and ■ Written statement of nutrition diagnosis.
Determination for Continuation of Care	Since the diagnosis step primarily involves naming and describing the problem, the determination for continuation of care seldom occurs at this step. Determination of the continuation of care is more appropriately made at an earlier or later point in the Nutrition Care Process.
	STEP 3. NUTRITION INTERVENTION
Basic Definition & Purpose	**"Nutrition Intervention"** is the third step of the Nutrition Care Process. An intervention is a specific set of activities and associated materials used to address the problem. Nutrition interventions are purposefully planned actions designed with the intent of changing a nutrition-related behavior, risk factor, environmental condition, or aspect of health status for an individual, target group, or the community at large. This step involves a) selecting, b) planning, and c) implementing appropriate actions to meet patient/client/groups' nutrition needs. The selection of nutrition interventions is driven by the nutrition diagnosis and provides the basis upon which outcomes are measured and evaluated. Dietetics professionals may actually do the interventions, or may include delegating or coordinating the nutrition care that others provide. All interventions must be based on scientific principles and rationale and, when available, grounded in a high level of quality research (evidence-based interventions). Dietetics professionals work collaboratively with the patient/client/group, family, or caregiver to create a realistic plan that has a good probability of positively influencing the diagnosis/problem. This client-driven process is a key element in the success of this step, distinguishing it from previous planning steps that may or may not have involved the patient/client/group to this degree of participation.
Data Sources/Tools for Interventions	■ Evidence-based nutrition guides for practice and protocols ■ Current research literature ■ Current consensus guidelines and recommendations from other professional organizations ■ Results of outcome management studies or Continuous Quality Index projects. ■ Current patient education materials at appropriate reading level and language ■ Behavior change theories (self-management training, motivational interviewing, behavior modification, modeling)
Nutrition Intervention Components	This step includes two distinct interrelated processes: **1. Plan the nutrition intervention** (formulate & determine a plan of action) ■ Prioritize the nutrition diagnoses based on severity of problem; safety; patient/client/group's need; likelihood that nutrition intervention will impact problem and patient/client/groups' perception of importance. ■ Consult ADA's *MNT Evidence-Based Guides for Practice* and other practice guides. These resources can assist dietetics professionals in identifying science-based ideal goals and selecting appropriate interventions for MNT. They list appropriate value(s) for control or improvement of the disease or conditions as defined and supported in the literature. ■ Determine patient-focused expected outcomes for each nutrition diagnosis. The expected outcomes are the desired change(s) to be achieved over time as a result of nutrition intervention. They are based on nutrition diagnosis; for example, increasing or decreasing laboratory values, decreasing blood pressure, decreasing weight, increasing use of stanols/sterols, or increasing fiber. Expected outcomes should be written in observable and measurable terms that are clear and concise. They should be patient/client/group-centered and need to be tailored to what is reasonable to the patient's circumstances and appropriate expectations for treatments and outcomes.

FIG 2 cont'd.

	■ Confer with patient/client/group, other caregivers or policies and program standards throughout planning step. ■ Define intervention plan (for example write a nutrition prescription, provide an education plan or community program, create policies that influence nutrition programs and standards). ■ Select specific intervention strategies that are focused on the etiology of the problem and that are known to be effective based on best current knowledge and evidence. ■ Define time and frequency of care including intensity, duration, and follow-up. ■ Identify resources and/or referrals needed. **2. Implement the nutrition intervention** (care is delivered and actions are carried out) ■ Implementation is the action phase of the nutrition care process. During implementation, dietetics professionals: □ Communicate the plan of nutrition care; □ Carry out the plan of nutrition care; and □ Continue data collection and modify the plan of care as needed. ■ Other characteristics that define quality implementation include: □ Individualize the interventions to the setting and client; □ Collaborate with other colleagues and health care professionals; □ Follow up and verify that implementation is occurring and needs are being met; and □ Revise strategies as changes in condition/response occurs.
Critical Thinking	Critical thinking is required to determine which intervention strategies are implemented based on analysis of the assessment data and nutrition diagnosis. The following types of critical thinking skills are especially needed in the intervention step: ■ Setting goals and prioritizing; ■ Transferring knowledge from one situation to another; ■ Defining the nutrition prescription or basic plan; ■ Making interdisciplinary connections; ■ Initiating behavioral and other interventions; ■ Matching intervention strategies with client needs, diagnoses, and values; ■ Choosing from among alternatives to determine a course of action; and ■ Specifying the time and frequency of care.
Documentation of Nutrition Interventions	Documentation is an on-going process that supports all of the steps in the Nutrition Care Process. Quality documentation of nutrition interventions should be relevant, accurate, and timely. It should also support further intervention or discharge from care. Changes in patient/client/group's level of understanding and food-related behaviors must be documented along with changes in clinical or functional outcomes to assure appropriate care/case management in the future. Inclusion of the following information would further describe quality documentation of this step: ■ Date and time; ■ Specific treatment goals and expected outcomes; ■ Recommended interventions, individualized for patient; ■ Any adjustments of plan and justifications; ■ Patient receptivity; ■ Referrals made and resources used; ■ Any other information relevant to providing care and monitoring progress over time; ■ Plans for follow-up and frequency of care; and ■ Rationale for discharge if appropriate.
Determination for Continuation of Care	If the patient/client/group has met intervention goals or is not at this time able/ready to make needed changes, the dietetics professional may include discharging the client from this episode of care as part of the planned intervention.
	STEP 4. NUTRITION MONITORING AND EVALUATION
Basic Definition & Purpose	**"Nutrition Monitoring and Evaluation"** is the fourth step of the Nutrition Care Process. *Monitoring* specifically refers to the review and measurement of the patient/client/group's status at a scheduled (preplanned) follow-up point with regard to the nutrition diagnosis, intervention plans/goals, and outcomes, whereas *Evaluation* is the systematic comparison of current findings with previous status, intervention goals, or a reference standard. Monitoring and evaluation use selected outcome indicators (markers) that are relevant to the patient/client/group's defined needs, nutrition diagnosis, nutrition goals, and disease state. Recommended times for follow-up, along with relevant outcomes to be monitored, can be found in ADA's Evidence Based Guides for Practice and other evidence-based sources. The purpose of monitoring and evaluation is to determine the degree to which progress is being made and goals or desired outcomes of nutrition care are being met. It is more than just "watching" what is happening, it requires an active commitment to measuring and recording the appropriate outcome indicators (markers) relevant to the nutrition diagnosis and intervention strategies. Data from this step are used to create an outcomes management system. Refer to Outcomes Management System in text.

FIG 2 cont'd.

	Progress should be monitored, measured, and evaluated on a planned schedule until discharge. Short inpatient stays and lack of return for ambulatory visits do not preclude monitoring, measuring, and evaluation. Innovative methods can be used to contact patients/clients to monitor progress and outcomes. Patient confidential self-report via mailings and telephone follow-up are some possibilities. Patients being followed in disease management programs can also be monitored for changes in nutritional status. Alterations in outcome indicators such as hemoglobin A1C or weight are examples that trigger reactivation of the nutrition care process.
Data Sources/Tools for Monitoring and Evaluation	■ Patient/client/group records ■ Anthropometric measurements, laboratory tests, questionnaires, surveys ■ Patient/client/group (or guardian) interviews/surveys, pretests, and posttests ■ Mail or telephone follow-up ■ ADA's *Evidence Based Guides for Practice* and other evidence-based sources ■ Data collection forms, spreadsheets, and computer programs
Types of Outcomes Collected	The outcome(s) to be measured should be directly related to the nutrition diagnosis and the goals established in the intervention plan. Examples include, but are not limited to: ■ Direct nutrition outcomes (knowledge gained, behavior change, food or nutrient intake changes, improved nutritional status); ■ Clinical and health status outcomes (laboratory values, weight, blood pressure, risk factor profile changes, signs and symptoms, clinical status, infections, complications); ■ Patient/client-centered outcomes (quality of life, satisfaction, self-efficacy, self-management, functional ability); and ■ Health care utilization and cost outcomes (medication changes, special procedures, planned/unplanned clinic visits, preventable hospitalizations, length of hospitalization, prevent or delay nursing home admission).
Nutrition Monitoring and Evaluation Components	This step includes three distinct and interrelated processes: **1. Monitor progress** ■ Check patient/client/group understanding and compliance with plan; ■ Determine if the intervention is being implemented as prescribed; ■ Provide evidence that the plan/intervention strategy is or is not changing patient/client/group behavior or status; ■ Identify other positive or negative outcomes; ■ Gather information indicating reasons for lack of progress; and ■ Support conclusions with evidence. **2. Measure outcomes** ■ Select outcome indicators that are relevant to the nutrition diagnosis or signs or symptoms, nutrition goals, medical diagnosis, and outcomes and quality management goals. ■ Use standardized indicators to: □ Increase the validity and reliability of measurements of change; and □ Facilitate electronic charting, coding, and outcomes measurement. **3. Evaluate outcomes** ■ Compare current findings with previous status, intervention goals, and/or reference standards.
Critical Thinking	The following types of critical thinking skills are especially needed in the monitoring and evaluation step: ■ Selecting appropriate indicators/measures; ■ Using appropriate reference standard for comparison; ■ Defining where patient/client/group is now in terms of expected outcomes; ■ Explaining variance from expected outcomes; ■ Determining factors that help or hinder progress; and ■ Deciding between discharge or continuation of nutrition care.
Documentation of Monitoring and Evaluation	Documentation is an on-going process that supports all of the steps in the Nutrition Care Process and is an integral part of monitoring and evaluation activities. Quality documentation of the monitoring and evaluation step should be relevant, accurate, and timely. It includes a statement of where the patient is now in terms of expected outcomes. Standardized documentation enables pooling of data for outcomes measurement and quality improvement purposes. Quality documentation should also include: ■ Date and time; ■ Specific indicators measured and results; ■ Progress toward goals (incremental small change can be significant therefore use of a Likert type scale may be more descriptive than a "met" or "not met" goal evaluation tool); ■ Factors facilitating or hampering progress; ■ Other positive or negative outcomes; and ■ Future plans for nutrition care, monitoring, and follow up or discharge.
Determination for Continuation of Care	Based on the findings, the dietetics professional makes a decision to actively continue care or discharge the patient/client/group from nutrition care (when necessary and appropriate nutrition care is completed or no further change is expected at this time). If nutrition care is to be continued, the nutrition care process cycles back as necessary to assessment, diagnosis, and/or intervention for additional assessment, refinement of the diagnosis and adjustment and/or reinforcement of the plan. If care does not continue, the patient may still be monitored for a change in status and reentry to nutrition care at a later date.

FIG 2 cont'd.

describing what dietetics professionals do is truly a paradigm shift. This new paradigm is more complete, takes in more possibilities, and explains observations better. Finally, it allows dietetics professionals to act in ways that are more likely to achieve the results that are desired and expected.

NUTRITION CARE MODEL

The Nutrition Care Model is a visual representation that reflects key concepts of each step of the Nutrition Care Process and illustrates the greater context within which the Nutrition Care Process is conducted. The model also identifies other factors that influence and impact on the quality of nutrition care provided. Refer to Figure 1 for an illustration of the model as described below:

- Central Core: Relationship between patient/client/group and dietetics professional;
- Nutrition Care Process: Four steps of the nutrition care process (Figure 2);
- Outer rings:
- Middle ring: Strengths and abilities that dietetics professionals bring to the process (dietetics knowledge, skills, and competencies; critical thinking, collaboration, and communication; evidence-based practice, and Code of Ethics) (32);
- Outer ring: Environmental factors that influence the process (practice settings, health care systems, social systems, and economics);
- Supporting Systems:
- Screening and Referral System as access to Nutrition Care; and
- Outcomes Management System as a means to provide continuous quality improvement to the process.

The model is intended to depict the relationship with which all of these components overlap, interact, and move in a dynamic manner to provide the best quality nutrition care possible.

Central to providing nutrition care is the relationship between the patient/client/group and the dietetics professional. The patient/client/groups' previous educational experiences and readiness to change influence this relationship. The education and training that dietetics professionals receive have very strong components devoted to interpersonal knowledge and skill building such as listening, empathy, coaching, and positive reinforcing.

The middle ring identifies abilities of dietetics professionals that are especially applicable to the Nutrition Care Process. These include the unique dietetics knowledge, skill, and competencies that dietetics professionals bring to the process, in addition to a well-developed capability for critical thinking, collaboration, and communication. Also in this ring is evidence-based practice that emphasizes that nutrition care must incorporate currently available scientific evidence, linking what is done (content) and how it is done (process of care). The Code of Ethics defines the ethical principles by which dietetics professionals should practice (33). Dietetics knowledge and evidence-based practice establish the Nutrition Care Process as unique to dietetics professionals; no other health care professional is qualified to provide nutrition care in this manner. However, the Nutrition Care Process is highly dependent on collaboration and integration within the health care team. As stated above, communication and participation within the health care team are critical for identification of individuals who are appropriate for nutrition care.

The outer ring identifies some of the environmental factors such as practice settings, health care systems, social systems, and economics. These factors impact the ability of the patient/client/group to receive and benefit from the interventions of nutrition care. It is essential that dietetics professionals assess these factors and be able to evaluate the degree to which they may be either a positive or negative influence on the outcomes of care.

Screening and Referral System

Because screening may or may not be accomplished by dietetics professionals, nutrition screening is a supportive system and *not* a step within the Nutrition Care Process. Screening is extremely important; it is an identification step that is outside the actual "care" and provides access to the Nutrition Care Process.

The Nutrition Care Process depends on an effective screening and/or referral process that identifies clients who would benefit from nutrition care or MNT. Screening is defined by the US Preventive Services Task Force as "those preventive services in which a test or standardized examination procedure is used to identify patients requiring special intervention" (34). The major requirements for a screening test to be considered effective are the following:

- Accuracy as defined by the following three components:
  - □ Specificity: Can it identify patients with a condition?
  - □ Sensitivity: Can it identify those who do not have the condition?
  - □ Positive and negative predictive; and
- Effectiveness as related to likelihood of positive health outcomes if intervention is provided.

Screening parameters need to be tailored to the population and to the nutrition care services to be provided. For example, the screening parameters identified for a large tertiary acute care institution specializing in oncology would be vastly different than the screening parameters defined for an ambulatory obstetrics clinic. Depending on the setting and institutional policies, the dietetics professional may or may not be directly involved in the screening process. Regardless of whether dietetics professionals are actively involved in conducting the screening process, they are accountable for providing input into the development of appropriate screening parameters to ensure that the screening process asks the right questions. They should also evaluate how effective the screening process is in terms of correctly identifying clients who require nutrition care.

In addition to correctly identifying clients who would benefit from nutrition care, a referral process may be necessary to ensure that the client has an identifiable method of being linked to dietetics professionals who will ultimately provide the nutrition care or medical nutrition therapy. While the nutrition screening and referral is not part of the Nutrition Care Process, it is a critical antecedent step in the overall system (35).

Outcomes Management System

An outcomes management system evaluates the effectiveness and efficiency of the entire process (assessment, diagnosis, interventions, cost, and others), whereas the fourth step of the process "nutrition monitoring and evaluations" refers to the evaluation of the patient/client/group's progress in achieving outcomes.

Because outcomes management is a system's commitment to effective and efficient care, it is depicted outside of the NCP. Outcomes management links care processes and resource utilization with outcomes. Through outcomes management, relevant data are collected and analyzed in a timely manner so that performance can be adjusted and improved. Findings are compared with such things as past levels of performance; organizational, regional, or national norms; and standards or benchmarks of optimal performance. Generally, this information is reported to providers, administrators, and payors/funders and may be part of administrative databases or required reporting systems.

It requires an infrastructure in which outcomes for the population served are routinely assessed, summarized, and reported. Health care organizations use complex information management systems to manage resources and track performance. Selected information documented throughout the nutrition care process is entered into these central information management systems and structured databases. Examples of centralized data systems in which nutrition care data should be included are the following:

- basic encounter documentation for billing and cost accounting;
- tracking of standard indicators for quality assurance and accreditation;
- pooling data from a large series of patients/clients/groups to determine outcomes; and
- specially designed studies that link process and outcomes to determine effectiveness and cost effectiveness of diagnostic and intervention approaches.

The major goal of outcomes management is to utilize collected data to improve the quality of care rendered in the future. Monitoring and evaluation data from individuals are pooled/aggregated for the purposes of professional accountability, outcomes management, and systems/processes improvement. Results from a large series of patients/clients can be used to determine the effectiveness of intervention strategies and the impact of nutrition care in improving the overall health of individuals and groups. The effects of well-monitored quality improvement initiatives should be reflected in measurable improvements in outcomes.

Outcomes management comprehensively evaluates the two parts of IOM's definition of quality: outcomes and process. Measuring the relationship between the process and the outcome is essential for quality improvement. To ensure that the quality of patient care is not compromised, the focus of quality improvement efforts should always be directed at the outcome of care (36-43).

FUTURE IMPLICATIONS

Impact on Coverage for Services

Quality-related issues are gaining in importance worldwide. Even though our knowledge base is increasing, the scientific evidence for most clinical practices in all of medicine is modest. So much of what is done in health care does *not* maximize quality or minimize cost (44). A standardized Nutrition Care Process is a necessary foundation tool for gathering valid and reliable data on how quality nutrition care provided by qualified dietetics professionals improves the overall quality of health care provided. Implementing ADA's Nutrition Care Process provides a framework for demonstrating that nutrition care improves outcomes by the following: (a) enhancing the health of individuals, groups, institutions, or health systems; (b) potentially reducing health care costs by decreasing the need for medications, clinic and hospital visits, and preventing or delaying nursing home admissions; and (c) serving as the basis for research, documenting the impact of nutrition care provided by dietetics professionals (45-47).

Developing Scopes and Practice Standards

The work group reviewed the questions raised by delegates regarding the role of the RD and DTR in the Nutrition Care Process. As a result of careful consideration of this important issue, it was concluded that describing the various types of tasks and responsibilities appropriate to each of these credentialed dietetics professionals was yet another professional issue beyond the intent and purpose of developing a standardized Nutrition Care Process.

A scope of practice of a profession is the range of services that the profession is authorized to provide. Scopes of practice, depending on the particular setting in which they are used, can have different applications. They can serve as a legal document for state certification/licensure laws or they might be incorporated into institutional policy and procedure guidelines or job descriptions. Professional scopes of practice should be based on the education, training, skills, and competencies of each profession (48).

As previously noted, a dietetics professional is a person who, by virtue of academic and clinical training and appropriate certification and/or licensure, is uniquely qualified to provide a comprehensive array of professional services relating to prevention and treatment of nutrition-related conditions. A Scope of Practice articulates the roles of the RD, DTR, and advanced-practice RD. Issues to be addressed for the future include the following: (a) the need for a common scope with specialized guidelines and (b) recognition of the rich diversity of practice vs exclusive domains of practice regulation.

Professional standards are "authoritative statements that describe performance common to the profession." As such, standards should encompass the following:

- articulate the expectations the public can have of a dietetics professional in any practice setting, domain, and/or role;
- expect and achieve levels of practice against which actual performance can be measured; and
- serve as a legal reference to describe "reasonable and prudent" dietetics practice.

The Nutrition Care Process effectively reflects the dietetics professional as the unique provider of nutrition care when it is consistently used as a systematic method to think critically and make decisions to provide safe and effective care. ADA's Nutrition Care Process will serve as a guide to develop scopes of practice and standards of practice (49,50). Therefore, the work group recommended that further work be done to use the Nutrition Care Process to describe roles and functions that can be included in scopes of practice. In May 2003, the Board of Directors of ADA established a Practice Definitions Task Force that will identify and differentiate the terms within the profession that need clarification for members, affiliates, and DPGs related to licensure, certification, practice acts, and advanced practice. This task force is also charged to clarify the scope of practice services, clinical privileges, and accountabilities provided by RDs/DTRs based on education, training, and experience.

Education of Dietetics Students

It will be important to review the current CADE Educational Standards to ensure that the language and level of expected competencies are consistent with the entry-level practice of the Nutrition Care Process. Further work by the Commission on Dietetic Registration (CDR) may need to be done to make revisions on the RD and DTR exams to evaluate entry-level competencies needed to practice nutrition care in this way. Revision of texts and other educational materials will also need to incorporate the key principles and steps of this new process (51).

Education and Credentialing of Members

Even though dietetics professionals currently provide nutrition care, this standardized Nutrition Care Process includes some new principles, concepts, and guidelines in each of its steps. This is especially true of steps 2 and 4 (Nutrition Diagnosis and Nutrition Monitoring and Evaluation). Therefore, the implications for education of dietetics professionals and their practice are great. Because a large number of dietetics professionals still are employed in health care systems, a comprehensive educational plan will be essential. A model to be considered when planning education is the one used to educate dietetics professionals on the Professional Development Portfolio (PDP) Process (52). Materials that could be used to provide members with the necessary knowledge and skills in this process could include but not be limited to the following:

- articles in the *Journal of the American Dietetic Association*;
- continuing professional education lectures and presentations at affiliate and national meetings;
- self-study materials; case studies, CD-ROM workbooks, and others;
- hands-on workshops and training programs;
- Web-based materials; and
- inclusion in the learning needs assessment and codes of the Professional Development Portfolio.

Through the development of this educational strategic plan, the benefits to dietetics professionals and other stakeholders will need to be a central theme to promote the change in practice that comes with using this process to provide nutrition care.

Evidence-Based Practice

The pressure to do more with less is dramatically affecting all of health care, including dietetics professionals. This pressure is forcing the health care industry to restructure to be more efficient and cost-effective in delivering care. It will require the use of evidenced-based practice to determine what practices are critical to support outcomes (53,54). The Nutrition Care Process will be invaluable as research is completed to evaluate the services provided by dietetics professionals (55). The Nutrition Care Process will provide the structure for developing the methodology and data collection in individual settings, and the practice-based research networks ADA is in the process of initiating.

Standardized Language

As noted in Step 2 (Nutrition Diagnosis), having a standard taxonomy for nutrition diagnosis would be beneficial. Work in the area of articulating the types of interventions used by dietetics professionals has already begun by the Definitions Work Group under the direction of ADA's Research Committee. Further work to define terms that are part of the Nutrition Care Process will need to continue. Even though the work group provided a list of terms relating to the definition and key concepts of the process, there are opportunities to articulate further terms that are consistently used in this process. The Board of Directors of ADA in May 2003 approved continuation and expansion of a task force to address a comprehensive system that includes a process for developing and validating standardized language for nutrition diagnosis, intervention, and outcomes.

SUMMARY

Just as maps are reissued when new roads are built and rivers change course, this Nutrition Care Process and Model reflects recent changes in the nutrition and health care environment. It provides dietetics professionals with the updated "road map" to follow the best path for high-quality patient/client/group-centered nutrition care.

References

1. American Dietetic Association Strategic Plan. Available at: http://eatright.org (member only section). Accessed June 2, 2003.
2. Wheeler D. *Understanding Variation: The Key to Managing Chaos*. 2nd ed. Knoxville, TN: SPC Press; 2000.
3. Shojania KG, Duncan BW, McDonald KM, Wachter RM. Making Health Care Safer: A Critical Analysis of Patient Safety Practices. Evidence Report/ Technology Assessment No. 43 (Prepared by the University of California at San Francisco-Stanford Evidence-based Practice Center under Contract No. 290-97-0013). Rockville, MD: Agency for Healthcare Research and Quality; 2001. Report No.: AHRQ Publication No. 01-E058.
4. Potter, Patricia A, Perry, Anne G. *Basic Nursing Theory and Practice*. 4th ed. St Louis: C.V. Mosby; 1998.
5. American Physical Therapy Association. *Guide to Physical Therapist Practice*. 2nd ed. Alexandria, VA; 2001.
6. The Guide to Occupational Therapy Practice. *Am J Occup Ther*. 1999;53:3. Available at http://nweb.pct.edu/homepage/student/NUNJOL02/ot%20 process.ppt. Accessed May 30, 2003.
7. Kohn KN, ed. *Medicare: A strategy for Quality Assurance, Volume I*. Committee to Design a Strategy for Quality Review and Assurance in Medicare. Washington, DC: Institute of Medicine. National Academy Press; 1990.
8. Kohn L, Corrigan J, Donaldson M, eds. *To Err Is Human: Building a Safer Health System*. Washington, DC: Committee on Quality of Health Care in America, Institute of Medicine. National Academy Press; 2000.
9. Institute of Medicine. *Crossing the Quality Chasm: A New Health System for the 21st Century*. Committee on Quality in Health Care in America. Rona Briere, ed. Washington, DC: National Academy Press; 2001.
10. Splett P. *Developing and Validating Evidence-Based Guides for Practice: A Tool Kit for Dietetics Professionals*. American Dietetic Association; 1999.
11. Endres JB. *Community Nutrition. Challenges and Opportunities*. Upper Saddle River, NJ: Prentice-Hall, Inc; 1999.
12. Splett P. Planning, Implementation and Evaluation of Nutrition Programs. In: Sharbaugh CO, ed. *Call to Action: Better Nutrition for Mothers, Children, and Families*. Washington, DC: National Center for Education in Maternal and Child Health (NCEMCH); 1990.
13. Batalden PB, Stoltz PA. A framework for the continual improvement of health care: Building and applying professional and improvement knowledge to test changes in daily work. *Jt Comm J Qual Improv*. 1993;19:424-452.
14. CADE Accreditation Handbook. Available at: http://www.eatright.com/ cade/standards.html. Accessed March 20, 2003.
15. Alfaro-LeFevre R. Nursing process overview. *Applying Nursing Process. Promoting Collaborative Care*. 5th ed. Lippincott; 2002.
16. Grant A, DeHoog S. *Nutrition Assessment Support and Management*. Northgate Station, WA; 1999.
17. Sandrick, K. Is nutritional diagnosis a critical step in the nutrition care process? *J Am Diet Assoc*. 2002;102:427-431.
18. King LS. What is a diagnosis? *JAMA*. 1967;202:154.
19. Doenges ME. *Application of Nursing Process and Nursing Diagnosis: An Interactive Text for Diagnostic Reasoning*, 3rd ed. Philadelphia, PA: FA Davis Co; 2000.
20. Gallagher-Alred C, Voss AC, Gussler JD. *Nutrition intervention and patient outcomes: a self-study manual*. Columbus, OH: Ross Products Division, Abbott Laboratories; 1995.
21. Splett P, Myers EF. A proposed model for effective nutrition care. *J Am Diet Assoc*. 2001;101:357-363.
22. Lacey K, Cross N. A problem-based nutrition care model that is diagnostic driven and allows for monitoring and managing outcomes. *J Am Diet Assoc*. 2002;102:578-589.
23. Brylinsky C. The Nutrition Care Process. In: Mahan K, Escott-Stump S,

eds. *Krause's Food, Nutrition and Diet Therapy*, 10th ed. Philadelphia, PA: W.B. Saunders Company; 2000:431-451.
24. Hammond MI, Guthrie HA. Nutrition clinic: An integrated component of an undergraduate curriculum. *J Am Diet Assoc.* 1985;85:594.
25. Final MNT Regulations. CMS-1169-FC. Federal Register, November 1, 2001. Department of Health and Human Services. 42 CFR Parts: 405, 410, 411, 414, and 415. Available at: http://cms.hhs.gov/physicians/pfs/cms1169fc.asp. Accessed June 27, 2003.
26. Commission on Dietetic Registration CDR Certifications and State Licensure. Available at: http://www.cdrnet.org/certifications/index.htm. Accessed May 30, 2003.
27. Medicare Coverage Policy Decision: Duration and Frequency of the Medical Nutrition Therapy *(MNT) Benefit* (No. CAG-00097N). Available at: http://cms.hhs.gov/ncdr/memo.asp?id=53. Accessed June 2, 2003.
28. American Dietetic Association Medical Nutrition Therapy Evidence-Based Guides For Practice. Hyperlipidemia Medical Nutrition Therapy Protocol. CD-ROM; 2001.
29. American Dietetic Association. Medical Nutrition Therapy Evidence-Based Guides for Practice. Nutrition Practice Guidelines for Type 1 and 2 Diabetes Mellitus CD-ROM; 2001.
30. American Dietetic Association. Medical Nutrition Therapy Evidence-Based Guides for Practice. Nutrition Practice Guidelines for Gestational Diabetes Mellitus. CD-ROM; 2001.
31. American Dietetic Association Medical Nutrition Therapy Evidence-Based Guides For Practice. Chronic Kidney Disease (non-dialysis) Medical Nutrition Therapy Protocol. CD-ROM; 2002.
32. Gates G. Ethics opinion: Dietetics professionals are ethically obligated to maintain personal competence in practice. *J Am Diet Assoc.* May 2003;103: 633-635.
33. Code of Ethics for the Profession of Dietetics. *J Am Diet Assoc.* 1999;99: 109-113.
34. US Preventive Services Task Force. Guide to Clinical Preventive Services, 2nd ed. Washington, DC: US Department of Health and Human Services, Office of Disease Prevention and Health Promotion; 1996.
35. Identifying patients at risk: ADA's definitions for nutrition screening and nutrition assessment. *J Am Diet Assoc.* 1994;94:838-839.
36. Donabedian A. *Explorations in Quality Assessment and Monitoring. Volume I: The Definition of Quality and Approaches to Its Assessment.* Ann Arbor, MI: Health Administration Press; 1980.
37. Carey RG, Lloyd RC. *Measuring Quality Improvement in Health Care: A Guide to Statistical Process Control Applications.* New York, Quality Resources; 1995.
38. Eck LH, Slawson DL, Williams R, Smith K, Harmon-Clayton K, Oliver D. A model for making outcomes research standard practice in clinical dietetics. *J Am Diet Assoc.* 1998;98:451-457.
39. Ireton-Jones CS, Gottschlich MM, Bell SJ. *Practice-Oriented Nutrition Research: An Outcomes Measurement Approach.* Gaithersburg, MD: Aspen Publishers, Inc.; 1998.
40. Kaye GL. *Outcomes Management: Linking Research to Practice.* Columbus, OH: Ross Products Division, Abbott Laboratories; 1996.
41. Splett P. *Cost Outcomes of Nutrition Intervention*, a *Three Part Monograph.* Evansville, IN: Mead Johnson & Company; 1996.
42. Plsekk P. 1994. Tutorial: Planning for data collection part I: Asking the right question. *Qual Manage Health Care.* 2:76-81.
43. American Dietetic Association. Israel D, Moore S, eds. *Beyond Nutrition Counseling: Achieving Positive Outcomes Through Nutrition Therapy.* 1996.
44. Stoline AM, Weiner JP. *The New Medical Marketplace: A Physician's Guide to the Health Care System in the 1990s.* Baltimore: Johns Hopkins Press; 1993.
45. Mathematica Policy Research, Inc. Best Practices in Coordinated Care March 22, 2000. Available at: http://www.mathematica-mpr.com/PDFs/bestpractices.pdf. Accessed February 22, 2003.
46. Bisognano MA. New skills needed in medical leadership: The key to achieving business results. *Qual Prog.* 2000;33:32-41.
47. Smith R. Expanding medical nutrition therapy: An argument for evidence-based practices. *J Am Diet Assoc.* 2003;103:313-314.
48. National Council of State Boards of Nursing Model Nursing Practice Act. Available at: http://www.ncsbn.org/public/regulation/nursing_practice_model_practice_act.htm. Accessed June 27, 2003.
49. Professional policies of the American College of Medical Quality (ACMQ). Available at: http://www.acmq.org/profess/list.htm. Accessed June 27, 2003.
50. American Dietetic Association. Standards of professional practice. *J Am Diet Assoc.* 1998;98:83-85.
51. O'Neil EH and the Pew Health Professions Commission. Recreating Health Professional Practice for a New Century. The Fourth Report of the Pew Health Professions Commission. Pew Health Professions Commission; December 1998.
52. Weddle DO. The professional development portfolio process: Setting goals for credentialing. *J Am Diet Assoc.* 2002;102:1439-1444.
53. Sackett DL, Rosenberg WMC, Gray J, Haynes RB, Richardson WS. Evidence based medicine: What it is and what it isn't. *Br Med J.* 1996;312: 71-72.
54. Myers EF, Pritchett E, Johnson EQ. Evidence-based practice guides vs. protocols: What's the difference? *J Am Diet Assoc.* 2001;101:1085-1090.
55. Manore MM, Myers EF. Research and the dietetics profession: Making a bigger impact. *J Am Diet Assoc.* 2003;103:108-112.

The Quality Management Committee Work Group developed the Nutrition Care Process and Model with input from the House of Delegates dialog (October 2002 HOD meeting, in Philadelphia, PA). The work group members are the following: Karen Lacey, MS, RD, Chair; Elvira Johnson, MS, RD; Kessey Kieselhorst, MPA, RD; Mary Jane Oakland, PhD, RD, FADA; Carlene Russell, RD, FADA; Patricia Splett, PhD, RD, FADA; Suzanne Bertocchi, DTR, and Tamara Otterstein, DTR; Ellen Pritchett, RD; Esther Myers, PhD, RD, FADA; Harold Holler, RD, and Karri Looby, MS, RD. The work group would like to extend a special thank you to Marion Hammond, MS, and Naomi Trossler, PhD, RD, for their assistance in development of the Nutrition Care Process and Model.

American Dietetic Association's Standardized Nutrition Language: Current Status

Introduction

Evidence-based dietetic practice relies on concise, consistent, and standardized terminology to create and retrieve digital sources of evidence.[1] This is essential for documenting nutrition diagnoses, interventions and outcomes in electronic health records. A task force of the American Dietetic Association (ADA) has begun to refine and disseminate standardized nutrition language. The language is built on the Nutrition Care Process and Model that maps quality nutrition care and outcomes, and recognizes several existing terminologies used by other health professions. This paper will describe the logic model for the development of the standardized nutrition language, the Nutrition Care Process it is built upon, and its current status.

The project goal is to support nutrition practice, education, research, and policy with data. It is assumed that practicing dietitians, educators, and researchers will use the standardized nutrition language to document care, aggregate data, and study the evidence. Standardized terminology will provide the foundation for developing a national dietitian care database.

The Nutrition Care Process

The ADA Nutrition Care Model workgroup published the Nutrition Care Process (NCP) and Model in August 2003.[2] It provides a definition of the NCP and describes its steps and framework. The NCP is "a systematic problem-solving method that dietetics professionals use to critically think and make decisions to address nutrition related problems and provide safe and effective quality nutrition care."[2, p1063] The four steps of the NCP, similar to those of other clinical professions, are: (a) Nutrition Assessment, (b) Nutrition Diagnosis, (c) Nutrition Intervention, and (d) Nutrition Monitoring and Evaluation. Allowing for the reality of an iterative and comprehensive clinical process, the NCP is not linear and it includes, but is not limited to, Medical Nutrition Therapy. Medical Nutrition Therapy is "nutritional diagnostic, therapy, and counseling services for the purpose of disease management, which are furnished by a registered dietitian or nutrition professional."[3] The context of the NCP and surrounding influences are captured in the Model framework.

Standardized terms are being developed for each step of the NCP. Nutrition Assessment is "a systematic process of obtaining, verifying, and interpreting data in order to make decisions about the nature and cause of nutrition-related problems."[2] The Nutrition Assessment includes signs and symptoms. Nutrition Diagnosis is "the identification and labeling that describes an actual occurrence, risk of, or potential for developing a nutritional problem that dietetics professionals are responsible for treating independently."[2]

Nutrition Interventions are "purposely planned actions designed with the intent of changing a nutrition-related behavior, risk factor, environmental condition, or aspect of health status for an individual, target group, or the community at large."[2,] Interventions are directed to influence the etiology or effects of a diagnosis. Nutrition Monitoring is "the review and measurement of the patient/client/group's status at a scheduled (preplanned) follow-up point with regard to the nutrition diagnosis, intervention plans/goals, and outcomes." Evaluation is "the systematic comparison of current findings with previous status, intervention goals, or a reference standard."[2] Evaluation may measure changes in signs and symptoms. The NCP steps guide the delivery of nutrition health services, education, and research and define categories for documentation of nutrition care.

Development: Comparison with Nursing

In comparison with the development of various nursing terminologies, the ADA nutrition language development has been much more rapid and centralized, due perhaps to comparatively smaller numbers of nutrition professionals and growing sophistication in information technology. Nursing terminology work began in the 1970s, including the North American Nursing Diagnosis Association (NANDA)[4] terminology, the Clinical Care Classification (CCC),[5] and others. NANDA is specific to nursing diagnoses, while the CCC addresses diagnoses, interventions, and outcomes. The Nursing Minimum Data Set,[6] which includes patient information, nursing diagnoses, nursing interventions, nursing outcomes, intensity level of nursing care, and a unique provider number, is an overarching framework for the various discrete nursing terminologies, similar to the NCP.

Portions of this document have been submitted for publication elsewhere

Why Does Dietetics Practice Need a Standardized Language?

There is currently no agreed upon mechanism by which dietetics professionals can communicate with each other or other health care professionals. Because of this lack of agreement, there is no easy way to classify, measure, and report on the outcomes of nutrition interventions in various patient populations. The Nutrition Care Process includes nutrition diagnosis and nutrition intervention as unique steps that provide registered dietitians a mechanism to consistently document and communicate the work of dietetics. There is currently no agreed upon terminology used in dietetics practice which makes it impossible to gather and aggregate data needed for research, education, and reimbursement justification via outcomes analysis.

Logic Model

A Logic Model is a simplified picture that describes the logical relationships among the resources invested, the activities that take place, and the benefits to be realized from the project and the environment in which the system/project occurs. With the help of an informatics consultant, the Standardized Language Task Force adopted a Project Logic Model that identifies the expected outcomes and impact of the Standardized Language of Dietetics. The goal of the dietetics terminology was seen to be "To provide data to foster nutrition practice, education, research, and policy."

Three time frames for evaluating the impact of the standardized language were agreed upon. The most immediate impacts were thought to include recommendations for coordination with existing terminologies, review of the structure of the dietetics terminology, to "cross-walk" the new terminology with existing terminologies to see if overlap exists, to review existing intervention terms, and to identify relevant policy issues regarding standardized nutrition language. Intermediate impacts were thought to include selection of a structure for the nutrition diagnostic labels, cross-walk of the intervention terms, to plan for generation of nutrition outcomes measures, create strategies for ongoing maintenance and updates of the language, to design and implement pilot testing of the standardized language, and to draft legislative and policy agendas. The ultimate impact was agreed to include delivery of quality, cost-effective nutrition care, national growth of nutrition care, inclusion of the standardized language in dietetics education and research, development of a national data warehouse for nutrition research, and support of policies designed to foster nutrition practice, education, and research.

Several assumptions were necessary in development of this logic model. The Task Force was in agreement that nutrition is an essential component of high quality health care. There was heightened awareness of the need for data to document the processes and outcomes of nutrition care in a variety of settings. It was also assumed that educators, practicing dietitians, and researchers would accept and implement the standardized language and would be willing to share data using the terminology for targeted studies and ultimately a national database.

Nutrition Diagnostic Labels

To date, over 60 Nutrition Diagnostic Labels have been defined by ADA work with focus groups, domain experts, and membership committees. Standardized Language Task Force members judged the match between nutrition diagnoses terms and similar terms listed in the National Library of Medicine's Unified Medical Language System (UMLS);[7] many terms have synonyms. One of the robust terminologies in the UMLS is SNOMED-CT.[8] Staff from SNOMED-CT were contacted to discuss the process of submitting nutrition terms.

The Nutrition Diagnostic Labels include 3 domains: Clinical, Behavioral-Environmental, and Intake. The domains, sub-classes, and specific diagnoses are defined in the most recent version, a summary of which follows.

DOMAIN: INTAKE

Defined as "actual problems related to intake of energy, nutrients, fluids, bioactive substances through oral diet or nutrition support (enteral or parenteral nutrition)"

Class: Caloric Energy Balance

Defined as "actual or estimated changes in energy (kcal)"

Class: Oral or Nutrition Support Intake

Defined as "actual or estimated food and beverage intake from oral diet or nutrition support compared with patient goal"

Class: Fluid Intake Balance

Defined as "actual or estimated fluid intake compared with patient goal"

Class: Bioactive Substances Balance

Defined as "actual or observed intake of bioactive substances, including single or multiple functional food components, ingredients, dietary supplements, alcohol"

Class: Nutrient Balance

Defined as "actual or estimated intake of specific nutrient groups or single nutrients as compared with desired levels"

Sub-Class: Fat and Cholesterol Balance

Sub-Class: Protein Balance

Sub-Class: Carbohydrate and Fiber Balance
Sub-Class: Vitamin Balance
Sub-Class: Mineral Balance

DOMAIN: CLINICAL

Defined as "nutritional findings/problems identified that relate to medical or physical conditions"

Class: Functional Balance
Defined as "change in physical or mechanical functioning that interferes with or prevents desired nutritional consequences"

Class: Biochemical Balance
Defined as "change in capacity to metabolize nutrients as a result of medications, surgery, or as indicated by altered lab values"

Class: Weight Balance
Defined as "chronic weight or changed weight status when compared with usual or desired body weight"

DOMAIN: BEHAVIORAL-ENVIRONMENTAL

Defined as "nutritional findings/problems identified that relate to knowledge, attitudes/beliefs, physical environment, or access to food and food safety"

Class: Knowledge and Beliefs
Defined as "actual knowledge and beliefs as reported, observed, or documented"

Class: Physical Activity Balance and Function
Defined as "actual physical activity, self-care, and quality of life problems as reported, observed or documented"

Class: Food Safety and Access
Defined as "actual problems with food access or food safety"

Problem-Etiology-Signs/Symptoms Statements

A Nutrition Diagnosis is best written as a PES statement pertaining to one patient/client or group, specific to one problem (P) and one etiology (E), and based on assessment of signs and symptoms (S).[2] Implementation of PES statements in clinical practice is being tested in two pilot studies by ADA members. Examples of PES statements are (a) "Overweight/obesity (problem) related to continued intake of high fat foods (etiology) resulting in ~300 extra kcal/day as evidenced by a BMI of 30 (sign/symptom), and (b) Impaired ability to prepare foods/meals (problem) related to fatigue (etiology) as evidenced by patient/client only consuming one meal per day." Interventions are often guided by the etiology of each problem. Signs and symptoms may provide measures to evaluate outcomes and the effectiveness of care. It is possible that the standardized terms for assessments will be considered relevant outcome measures.

Nutrition Interventions

Following principles for standardized terminologies,[9] the ADA has begun to identify and define Nutrition Intervention terms. A Task Force meeting in February 2005 identified categories of interventions including: Treatments/Procedures, Education, Counseling, and Referral/Coordination. These categories are similar to those in nursing terminologies but differing by not including monitoring/assessment as an intervention, which is a separate step in the Nutrition Care Process. Synonyms to the intervention terms will be searched in the UMLS and domain experts will judge the extent of the matches. The Nutrition Intervention Labels will be submitted SNOMED-CT or other existing coding system that will be included in the UMLS.

Future Work

Definition of Nutrition Assessment terms and their relationship with Outcome terms is planned. In addition, activities to communicate the standardized language to educators, administrators, clinicians, and researchers are planned. The ADA believes that consistent standardized terminology will improve patient care by enhancing the education, practice, and research of nutrition professionals. The use of standardized nutrition language by nutrition professionals in the United States is in synch with similar international efforts.

References

1. Bakken S. An informatics infrastructure is essential for evidence-based practice. *J Am Med Inform Assoc.* 2001;8:199-201.
2. Lacey K, Pritchett E. Nutrition care process and model: ADA adopts road map to quality care and outcomes management. *J Am Diet Assoc.* 2003;103:1061-72.
3. Final Medical Nutrition Therapy regulations. CMS-1169-FC. *Federal Register*, Nov.1, 2001. DHHS 42 CFR Parts: 405, 410, 411, 414, and 415. Available at:http://cms.hhs.gov/physicians/pfs/cms1169fc.asp? Accessed: March 7, 2005.
4. North American Nursing Diagnosis Association. Available at: http://www.nanda.org. Accessed Mar. 7, 2005.
5. Saba V. Clinical Care Classification System. Available at http://www.sabacare.com. Accessed March 7, 2005.
6. Werley H, Lang NM. *Identification of the Nursing Minimum Data Set.* New York:NY: Springer; 1988.

7. National Library of Medicine. Unified Medical Language System. 2005. Available at: http://www.nlm.nih.gov/research/umls/umlsmain.html. Accessed March 7, 2005.

8. College of American Pathologists. SNOMED International Clinical Terms. Available at http://www.snomed.org/. Accessed March 7, 2005.

9. Cimino JJ. Desiderata for controlled medical vocabularies in the twenty-first century. *Meth Inform Med*; 1998;37:394-403.

Portions of this document have been submitted for publication elsewhere

Introduction to Nutrition Diagnoses/Problems:
The New Component of the Nutrition Care Process

Introduction

The ADA has embarked on an extensive project to identify and define nutrition diagnoses/problems for the profession of dietetics. This standardized language of nutrition diagnoses/problems is an integral component in the Nutrition Care Process, a process designed to improve the consistency and quality of individualized patient/client care and the predictability of the patient/client outcomes. In fact, several other allied professional, including nursing, physical therapy, and occupational therapy, utilize defined care processes (1).

Not only will creating this standard language help dietetic professionals better document their nutrition care, it will serve to help achieve Association strategic goals of promoting demand for dietetic professionals and help them be more competitive in the market place. It will also provide a minimum data set and common data elements for future research that includes services of dietetic professionals.

ADA's Standardized Language Task Force developed a conceptual framework for the standardized nutrition language and identified the nutrition diagnoses/problems. The framework outlines the domains within which the diagnoses/problems would fall and the flow of the nutrition care process in relation to the continuum of health, disease and disability. Sixty-two diagnoses/problems have been identified. A worksheet has been developed for each diagnosis/problem and expert has been incorporated.

The methodology for developing sets of terms such as these includes systematically collecting data from multiple sources simultaneously. We collected data from a selected group of dietitians prior to starting the project (from recognized ADA leaders and award winners), from the 12 member task force during the development, from several small group discussions (community, ambulatory, acute care, and long term care), and from expert researcher reviewers.

The methodology for continued development and refinement of these terms has been identified. As with the ongoing updating of the American Medical Association Current Procedural Terminology (CPT) codes, these will also be published on an annual basis. The process to submit your suggested changes is included in this packet. In addition, the terms have been included in one ongoing research project in an ambulatory setting. A second descriptive research study identifying the use of the terms will be planned and conducted through the Dietetics Practice Based Research Network in 2005-2006. As each of the research studies is completed, their findings will be incorporated into future versions of these terms. Future iterations and changes to the diagnoses/problems and the worksheets are expected as this standard language evolves. Once the initial research is completed we will formally submit these terms to become part of nationally recognized health care databases. We have already begun the dialogue with these groups to let them know the direction that we are headed and to keep them appraised of our progress.

Nutrition Care Process and Nutrition Diagnosis

ADA's new nutrition care process for the profession has four steps—nutrition assessment, nutrition diagnosis, nutrition intervention, and nutrition monitoring and evaluation (1). Textbooks often describe nutrition assessment in detail and then move directly into intervention or therapy. **Nutrition diagnosis** is a critical step between assessment and intervention. The nutrition diagnosis is the identification and labeling of the specific nutrition problem that dietetics professionals are responsible for treating independently.

Naming the nutrition diagnosis provides a way to document the link between nutrition assessment and nutrition intervention and set realistic and measurable expected outcomes for each patient/client. Identifying the diagnosis also assists practitioners in establishing priorities when planning an individual patient/client's nutrition care.

Nutrition diagnosis differs from medical diagnosis. Medical diagnosis is a disease or pathology of specific organs or body systems (e.g., diabetes) and does not change as long as the condition exists. A nutrition diagnosis may be temporary, altering as the patient/client's response changes (e.g., excessive carbohydrate intake).

Categorization of the Nutrition Diagnoses

The sixty-two nutrition diagnoses/problems have been given labels that are clustered into three domains: intake, clinical, and behavioral-environmental. Each domain represents unique characteristics that contribute to nutritional health. Within each domain are classes and, in some cases, sub-classes of diagnoses. A definition of each follows:

The **Intake** domain lists actual problems related to intake of energy, nutrients, fluids, bioactive substances through oral diet, or nutrition support (enteral or parenteral nutrition.)

Class: Caloric Energy Balance (1)—Actual or estimated changes in energy (kcal).
Class: Oral or Nutrition Support Intake (2)—Actual or estimated food and beverage intake from oral diet or nutrition support compared with patient/client's goal.
Class: Fluid Intake Balance (3)—Actual or estimated fluid intake compared with patient/client's goal.
Class: Bioactive Substances Balance (4)—Actual or observed intake of bioactive substances, including single or multiple functional food components, ingredients, dietary supplements, and alcohol.
Class: Nutrient Balance (5)—Actual or estimated intake of specific nutrient groups or single nutrients as compared with desired levels.

- Sub-Class: Fat and Cholesterol Balance (51)
- Sub-Class: Protein Balance (52)
- Sub-Class: Carbohydrate and Fiber Balance (53)
- Sub-Class: Vitamin Balance (54)
- Sub-Class: Mineral Balance (55)

The **Clinical** domain is nutritional findings/problems identified that relate to medical or physical conditions.

Class: Functional Balance (1)—Change in physical or mechanical function that interferes with or prevents desired nutritional consequences.

Class: Biochemical Balance (2)—Change in the capacity to metabolize nutrients as a result of medications, surgery, or as indicated by altered lab values.
Class: Weight Balance (3)—Chronic weight or changed weight status when compared with usual or desired body weight.

The **Behavioral-Environmental** domain includes nutritional findings/problems identified that relate to knowledge, attitudes/beliefs, physical environment, access to food, and food safety.

Class: Knowledge and Beliefs (1)—Actual knowledge and beliefs as reported, observed, or documented.
Class: Physical Activity Balance and Function (2)—Actual physical activity, self-care, and quality of life problems as reported, observed, or documented.
Class: Food Safety and Access (3)—Actual problems with food access or food safety.

Examples of nutrition diagnoses and their definitions include:

INTAKE DOMAIN ▪ Caloric Energy Balance

Inadequate energy intake NI-1.4	Energy intake that is less than energy expenditure or recommended levels. Exception: when the goal is for the client to lose weight or during end of life care.

CLINICAL DOMAIN ▪ Functional Balance

Swallowing difficulty NC-1.1	Impaired movement of food and liquid from the mouth to the stomach.

BEHAVIORAL-ENVIRONMENTAL DOMAIN ▪ Knowledge and Beliefs

Not ready for diet/lifestyle change NB-1.3	Lack of perceived value of nutrition-related care benefits compared to consequences or effort required to making the change; inconsistencies with other value structure/purpose; antecedent to behavior change.

Nutrition Diagnosis Statements (or PES)

Whenever possible, a nutrition diagnosis statement is written in the *PES* format that states the **problem** (P), the **etiology** (E), and the **signs/symptoms** (S).

Examples

▪ Swallowing difficulty (problem) related to stroke (etiology) as evidenced by coughing following drinking of thin liquids (sign/symptoms).

▪ Inadequate energy intake (problem) related to lack of financial resources to purchase sufficient food (etiology) as evidenced by weight loss of 6 pounds in the last 2 months (signs/symptoms).

Nutrition Diagnosis Worksheet

A worksheet has been developed for each diagnosis. It contains four distinct components: nutrition diagnosis label, definition of nutrition diagnosis label, etiology, and signs/symptoms. These worksheets will assist practitioners with consistently and correctly utilizing the nutrition diagnoses. Below is a description of the four components of the worksheet.

The **Problem or Nutrition Diagnosis Label** describes alterations in the patient/client's nutrition status that dietetics professionals are responsible for treating independently. Nutrition diagnosis differs from medical diagnosis in that a nutrition diagnosis changes as the patient/client response changes. The medical diagnosis does not change as long as the disease or condition exists. A nutrition diagnosis allows the dietetics professional to identify realistic and measurable outcomes, formulate interventions, and monitor and evaluate change.

The **Definition of Nutrition Diagnosis Label** briefly describes the Nutrition Diagnosis Label to differentiate a discrete problem area.

The **Etiology (Cause/Contributing Risk Factors)** are those factors contributing to the existence of, or maintenance of pathophysiological, psychosocial, situational, developmental, cultural, and/or environmental problems. It is linked to the diagnosis label by the words "related to."

The **Signs/Symptoms (Defining Characteristics)** consist of subjective and/or objective data used to determine whether the patient/client has the nutrition diagnosis specified. These are the signs and symptoms gathered through nutrition assessment. It is linked to the etiology by the words "as evidenced by."

Organization of Data in Signs/Symptoms (Defining Characteristics)

Dietetics professionals use clinical judgment to determine the nutrition diagnosis based on data collected from the first step of the nutrition care process: nutrition assessment. Therefore, the items listed in the signs/symptoms (defining characteristics) are organized according to nutrition assessment category.

Nutrition assessment is the systematic process for obtaining, verifying, and interpreting data needed to make decisions about the nature and cause of the nutrition-related problem. The process of nutrition assessment consists of collecting biochemical data, anthropometric measurements, physical examination findings, food/nutrition history, and client history. On the nutrition diagnosis worksheet, the signs/symptoms are classified by nutrition assessment categories.

Biochemical Data include laboratory data, for example, electrolytes, glucose, hemoglobin A1C, thyroid, and lipid panel.

Anthropometric Measurements include, for instance, height, weight, body mass index (BMI), growth rate, and rate of weight change.

Nutrition-Focused Physical Examination includes oral health, general physical appearance, muscle and subcutaneous fat wasting, and affect.

Food and Nutrition History consists of four areas: Food consumption, nutrition and health awareness and management, physical activity and exercise, and food availability.

> Food consumption may include factors such as, food and nutrient intake, meal and snack patterns, environmental cues to eating, and current diets and/or food modifications.
>
> Nutrition and health awareness and management includes, for example, knowledge and beliefs about nutrition recommendations, self-monitoring/management practices, and past nutrition counseling and education.
>
> Physical activity and exercise consists of activity patterns, amount of sedentary time (e.g., TV, phone, computer), and exercise intensity, frequency, and duration.
>
> Food availability encompasses factors such as, food planning, purchasing, preparation abilities and limitations, food safety practices, food/nutrition program utilization, and food insecurity.

Client History consists of four areas: Medication and supplement history, social history, medical/health history, and personal history.

> Medication and supplement history includes, for instance, prescription and over the counter drugs, herbal and dietary supplements, and illegal drugs.
>
> Social history may include such items as socioeconomic status, social and medical support, cultural and religious beliefs, housing situation, and social isolation/connection.
>
> Medical/health history includes chief nutrition complaint, present/past illness, disease or complication risk, family medical history, mental/emotional health, and cognitive abilities.
>
> Personal history consists of factors including age, occupation, role in family, and education level.

Summary

Nutrition diagnosis is the critical link in the nutrition care process between assessment and intervention. Interventions can then be clearly targeted to address either the etiology or signs and symptoms of the specific nutrition diagnosis/problem identified. Using a standardized terminology for identifying the nutrition diagnosis/problem will make one aspect of the critical thinking that dietetics professionals do visible to other professionals as well as provide a clear method of communicating among dietetics professionals. Implementation of a standard language throughout the profession, with tools to assist practitioners, will make this bold initiative a success. Ongoing input is critical as the standardized language is created to ensure a proper foundation for its future implementation.

Reference

1. Lacey K, Pritchett E. Nutrition care process and model: ADA adopts road map to quality care and outcomes management. *J Am Diet Assoc.* 2003;103:1061-1072.

NUTRITION DIAGNOSTIC TERMINOLOGY

INTAKE NI

Defined as "actual problems related to intake of energy, nutrients, fluids, bioactive substances through oral diet or nutrition support"

Caloric Energy Balance (1)

Defined as "actual or estimated changes in energy (kcal)"

- ☐ Hypermetabolism (*Increased energy needs*) NI-1.1
- ☐ Increased energy expenditure NI-1.2
- ☐ Hypometabolism (*Decreased energy needs*) NI-1.3
- ☐ Inadequate energy intake NI-1.4
- ☐ Excessive energy intake NI-1.5

Oral or Nutrition Support Intake (2)

Defined as "actual or estimated food and beverage intake from oral diet or nutrition support compared with patient goal"

- ☐ Inadequate oral food/beverage intake NI-2.1
- ☐ Excessive oral food/beverage intake NI-2.2
- ☐ Inadequate intake from enteral/parenteral nutrition infusion NI-2.3
- ☐ Excessive intake from enteral/parenteral nutrition NI-2.4
- ☐ Inappropriate infusion of enteral/parenteral nutrition (use with caution) NI-2.5

Fluid Intake (3)

Defined as "actual or estimated fluid intake compared with patient goal"

- ☐ Inadequate fluid intake NI-3.1
- ☐ Excessive fluid intake NI-3.2

Bioactive Substance Intake (4)

Defined as "actual or observed intake of bioactive substances, including single or multiple functional food components, ingredients, dietary supplements, alcohol"

- ☐ Inadequate bioactive substance intake NI-4.1
- ☐ Excessive bioactive substance intake NI-4.2
- ☐ Excessive alcohol intake NI-4.3

Nutrient Intake (5)

Defined as "actual or estimated intake of specific nutrient groups or single nutrients as compared with desired levels"

- ☐ Increased nutrient needs (*specify*) ____________ NI-5.1
- ☐ Evident protein-energy malnutrition NI-5.2
- ☐ Inadequate protein-energy intake NI-5.3
- ☐ Decreased nutrient needs (*specify*) ____________ NI-5.4
- ☐ Imbalance of nutrients NI-5.5

Fat and Cholesterol (51)

- ☐ Inadequate fat intake NI-51.1
- ☐ Excessive fat intake NI-51.2
- ☐ Inappropriate intake of food fats (*specify*) ____________ NI-51.3

Protein (52)

- ☐ Inadequate protein intake NI-52.1
- ☐ Excessive protein intake NI-52.2
- ☐ Inappropriate intake of amino acids (*specify*) ____________ NI-52.3

Carbohydrate and Fiber (53)

- ☐ Inadequate carbohydrate intake NI-53.1
- ☐ Excessive carbohydrate intake NI-53.2
- ☐ Inappropriate intake of types of carbohydrate (*specify*) ____________ NI-53.3
- ☐ Inconsistent carbohydrate intake NI-53.4
- ☐ Inadequate fiber intake NI-53.5
- ☐ Excessive fiber intake NI-53.6

Vitamin (54)

- ☐ Inadequate vitamin intake (*specify*) NI-54.1
- ☐ Excessive vitamin intake (*specify*) NI-54.2
  - ☐ A ☐ C
  - ☐ Thiamin ☐ D
  - ☐ Riboflavin ☐ E
  - ☐ Niacin ☐ K
  - ☐ Folate ☐ Other ______

Mineral (55)

- ☐ Inadequate mineral intake (*specify*) NI-55.1
  - ☐ Calcium ☐ Iron
  - ☐ Potassium ☐ Zinc
  - ☐ Other ____________
- ☐ Excessive mineral intake (*specify*) NI-55.2
  - ☐ Calcium ☐ Iron
  - ☐ Potassium ☐ Zinc
  - ☐ Other ____________

CLINICAL NC

Defined as "nutritional findings/problems identified as related to medical or physical conditions"

Functional (1)

Defined as "change in physical or mechanical functioning that interferes with or prevents desired nutritional consequences"

- ☐ Swallowing difficulty NC-1.1
- ☐ Chewing (*masticatory*) difficulty NC-1.2
- ☐ Breastfeeding difficulty NC-1.3
- ☐ Altered GI function NC-1.4

Biochemical (2)

Defined as "change in capacity to metabolize nutrients as a result of medications, surgery, or as indicated by altered lab values"

- ☐ Impaired nutrient utilization NC-2.1
- ☐ Altered nutrition-related laboratory values (*specify*) ____________ NC-2.2
- ☐ Food-medication interaction NC-2.3

Weight (3)

Defined as "chronic weight or changed weight status when compared with usual or desired body weight"

- ☐ Underweight NC-3.1
- ☐ Involuntary weight loss NC-3.2
- ☐ Overweight/obesity NC-3.3
- ☐ Involuntary weight gain NC-3.4

BEHAVIORAL-ENVIRONMENTAL NB

Defined as "nutritional findings/problems identified as related to knowledge, attitudes/beliefs, physical environment, or food supply and safety"

Knowledge and Beliefs (1)

Defined as "actual knowledge and beliefs as reported or documented"

- ☐ Food, nutrition, and nutrition-related knowledge deficit NB-1.1
- ☐ Harmful beliefs/attitudes about food or nutrition-related topics (use with caution) NB-1.2
- ☐ Not ready for diet/lifestyle change NB-1.3
- ☐ Self-monitoring deficit NB-1.4
- ☐ Disordered eating pattern NB-1.5
- ☐ Limited adherence to nutrition-related recommendations NB-1.6
- ☐ Undesirable food choices NB-1.7

Physical Activity and Function (2)

Defined as "actual physical activity, self-care, and quality of life problems as reported, observed, or documented"

- ☐ Physical inactivity NB-2.1
- ☐ Excessive exercise NB-2.2
- ☐ Inability or lack of desire to manage self-care NB-2.3
- ☐ Impaired ability to prepare foods/meals NB-2.4
- ☐ Poor nutrition quality of life NB-2.5
- ☐ Self-feeding difficulty NB-2.6

Food Safety and Access (3)

Defined as "actual problems with food access or food safety"

- ☐ Intake of unsafe food NB-3.1
- ☐ Limited access to food NB-3.2

Date Identified	Date Resolved

#1 Problem ____

Etiology ____

Signs/Symptoms ____

#2 Problem ____

Etiology ____

Signs/Symptoms ____

#3 Problem ____

Etiology ____

Signs/Symptoms ____

NUTRITION DIAGNOSIS TERMS AND DEFINITIONS

Nutrition Diagnostic Term	Term Number	Definition of Diagnostic Term	Reference Sheet Page Numbers
DOMAIN: INTAKE **Defined as "actual problems related to intake of energy, nutrients, fluids, bioactive substances through oral diet or nutrition support (enteral or parenteral nutrition)"**	NI		
Class: Caloric Energy Balance (1) ***Defined as "actual or estimated changes in energy (kcal)"***			
Hypermetabolism (Increased energy needs)	NI-1.1	Resting metabolic rate (RMR) above predicted requirements due to stress, trauma, injury, sepsis, or disease. Note: RMR is the sum of metabolic processes of active cell mass related to the maintenance of normal body functions and regulatory balance during rest.	32-33
Increased energy expenditure	NI-1.2	Resting metabolic rate (RMR) above predicted requirements due to body composition, medications, endocrine, neurologic, or genetic changes. Note: RMR is the sum of metabolic processes of active cell mass related to the maintenance of normal body functions and regulatory balance during rest.	34
Hypometabolism (Decreased energy needs)	NI-1.3	Resting metabolic rate (RMR) below predicted requirements due to body composition, medications, endocrine, neurologic, or genetic changes	35-36
Inadequate energy intake	NI-1.4	Energy intake that is less than energy expenditure, established reference standards, or recommendations based upon physiological needs. Exception: when the goal is weight loss or	37-38

NUTRITION DIAGNOSIS TERMS AND DEFINITIONS

		during end of life care.	
Excessive energy intake	NI-1.5	Caloric intake that exceeds energy expenditure, established reference standards, or recommendations based upon physiological needs. Exception: when weight gain is desired.	39-40
Class: Oral or Nutrition Support Intake (2) ***Defined as "actual or estimated food and beverage intake from oral diet or nutrition support compared with patient goal"***			
Inadequate oral food/beverage intake	NI-2.1	Oral food/beverage intake that is less than established reference standards or recommendations based upon physiological needs. Exception: when recommendation is weight loss or during end of life care.	41-42
Excessive oral food/beverage intake	NI-2.2	Oral food/beverage intake that exceeds energy expenditure, established reference standards, or recommendations based upon physiological needs. Exception: when weight gain is desired.	43-44
Inadequate intake from enteral/parenteral nutrition infusion	NI-2.3	Enteral or parenteral infusion that provides fewer calories or nutrients compared to established reference standards or recommendations based upon physiological needs. Exception: when recommendation is for weight loss or during end of life care.	45-46
Excessive intake from enteral/parenteral nutrition	NI-2.4	Enteral or parenteral infusion that provides more calories or nutrients compared to established reference standards or recommendations based upon physiological needs	47-48
Inappropriate infusion of enteral/parenteral nutrition USE WITH CAUTION ONLY AFTER DISCUSSION WITH OTHER MEMBERS OF THE HEALTH CARE TEAM	NI-2.5	Enteral or parenteral infusion that provides either fewer or more calories and/or nutrients or is of the wrong composition or type, is not warranted because the patient is able to tolerate an enteral intake, or is unsafe because of the potential for sepsis or other complications	49-50

NUTRITION DIAGNOSIS TERMS AND DEFINITIONS

Class: Fluid Intake (3) ***Defined as "actual or estimated fluid intake compared with patient goal"***			
Inadequate fluid intake	NI-3.1	Lower intake of fluid containing foods or substances compared to established reference standards or recommendations based upon physiological needs	51-52
Excessive fluid intake	NI-3.2	Higher intake of fluid compared to established reference standards or recommendations based upon physiological needs	53-54
Class: Bioactive Substances (4) ***Defined as "actual or observed intake of bioactive substances, including single or multiple functional food components, ingredients, dietary supplements, alcohol"***			
Inadequate bioactive substance intake	NI-4.1	Lower intake of bioactive substances containing foods or substances compared to established reference standards or recommendations based upon physiological needs	55-56
Excessive bioactive substance intake	NI-4.2	Higher intake of bioactive substances other than traditional nutrients, such as functional foods, bioactive food components, dietary supplements, food concentrates compared to established reference standards or recommendations based upon physiological needs	57-58
Excessive alcohol intake	NI-4.3	Intake above the suggested limits for alcohol	59-60
Class: Nutrient (5) ***Defined as "actual or estimated intake of specific nutrient groups or single nutrients as compared with desired levels"***			
Increased nutrient needs (specify)	NI-5.1	Increased need for a specific nutrient compared to established reference standards or recommendations based upon	61-62

		physiological needs	
Evident protein-energy malnutrition	NI-5.2	Inadequate intake of protein and/or energy	63-64
Inadequate protein-energy intake	NI-5.3	Inadequate intake of protein and/or energy compared to established reference standards or recommendations based upon physiological needs of short or recent duration	65-66
Decreased nutrient needs (specify)	NI-5.4	Decreased need for a specific nutrient compared to established reference standards or recommendations based upon physiological needs	67-68
Imbalance of nutrients	NI-5.5	An undesirable combination of ingested nutrients, such that the amount of one nutrient ingested interferes with or alters absorption and/or utilization of another nutrient	69-70
Sub-Class: Fat and Cholesterol (51)			
Inadequate fat intake	NI-51.1	Lower fat intake compared to established reference standards or recommendations based upon physiological needs. Exception: when recommendation is for weight loss or during end of life care.	71
Excessive fat intake	NI-51.2	Higher fat intake compared to established reference standards or recommendations based upon physiological needs	72-73
Inappropriate intake of food fats (specify)	NI-51.3	Intake of wrong type or quality of food fats compared to established reference standards or recommendations based upon physiological needs	74-75
Sub-Class: Protein (52)			
Inadequate protein intake	NI-52.1	Lower intake of protein containing foods or substances compared to established reference standards or recommendations based upon physiological needs	76
Excessive protein intake	NI-52.2	Intake above the recommended level and/or type of protein compared to established reference standards or	77-78

		recommendations based upon physiological needs	
Inappropriate intake of amino acids (specify)	NI-52.3	Intake that is more or less than recommended level and/or type of amino acids compared to established reference standards or recommendations based upon physiological needs	78-80
Sub-Class: Carbohydrate and Fiber (53)			
Inadequate carbohydrate intake	NI-53.1	Lower intake of carbohydrate-containing foods or substances compared to established reference standards or recommendations based upon physiological needs	81
Excessive carbohydrate intake	NI-53.2	Intake above the recommended level and type of carbohydrate compared to established reference standards or recommendations based upon physiological needs	82-83
Inappropriate intake of types of carbohydrate (specify)	NI-53.3	Intake or the type or amount of carbohydrate that is above or below the established reference standards or recommendations based upon physiological needs	84-85
Inconsistent carbohydrate intake	NI-53.4	Inconsistent timing of carbohydrate intake throughout the day, day to day, or a pattern of carbohydrate intake that is not consistent with recommended pattern based upon physiological needs	86-87
Inadequate fiber intake	NI-53.5	Lower intake of fiber-containing foods or substances compared to established reference standards or recommendations based upon physiological needs	88-89
Excessive fiber intake	NI-53.6	Higher intake of fiber-containing foods or substances compared to recommendations based upon patient/client condition	90-91
Sub-Class: Vitamin (54)			
Inadequate vitamin intake (specify)	NI-54.1	Lower intake of vitamin-containing foods or substances compared to established reference standards or recommendations based upon physiological needs	92-94

Excessive vitamin intake (specify)	NI-54.2	Higher intake of vitamin containing foods or substances compared to established reference standards or recommendations based upon physiological needs	95-96
Sub-Class: Mineral (55)			
Inadequate mineral intake (specify)	NI-55.1	Lower intake of mineral containing foods or substances compared to established reference standards or recommendations based upon physiological needs	97-98
Excessive mineral intake (specify)	NI-55.2	Higher intake of mineral from foods, supplements, medications or water, compared to established reference standards or recommendations based upon physiological needs	99-100
DOMAIN: CLINICAL **Defined as "nutritional findings/problems identified that relate to medical or physical conditions"**	NC		
Class: Functional (1) ***Defined as "change in physical or mechanical functioning that interferes with or prevents desired nutritional consequences"***			
Swallowing difficulty	NC-1.1	Impaired movement of food and liquid from the mouth to the stomach	101
Chewing (masticatory) difficulty	NC-1.2	Impaired ability to manipulate or masticate food for swallowing	102-104
Breastfeeding difficulty	NC-1.3	Inability to sustain nutrition through breastfeeding	105-106
Altered GI function	NC-1.4	Changes in ability to digest or absorb nutrients	107-108
Class: Biochemical (2) ***Defined as "change in capacity to metabolize nutrients as a result of***			

medications, surgery, or as indicated by altered lab values"			
Impaired nutrient utilization	NC-2.1	Changes in ability to absorb or metabolize nutrients and bioactive substances	109-110
Altered nutrition-related laboratory values	NC-2.2	Changes in ability to eliminate by-products of digestive and metabolic processes	111-112
Food-medication interaction	NC-2.3	Undesirable/harmful interaction(s) between food and over the counter (OTC) medications, prescribed medications, herbals, botanicals, and/or dietary supplements that diminishes, enhances, or alters effect of nutrients and/or medications	113-114
Class: Weight (3) ***Defined as "chronic weight or changed weight status when compared with usual or desired body weight"***			
Underweight	NC-3.1	Low body weight compared to established reference standards or recommendations	115-116
Involuntary weight loss	NC-3.2	Decrease in body weight that is not planned or desired	117-118
Overweight/obesity	NC-3.3	Increased adiposity compared to established reference standards or recommendations	119-120
Involuntary weight gain	NC-3.4	Weight gain above that which is desired or expected	121-122
DOMAIN: BEHAVIORAL-ENVIRONMENTAL **Defined as "nutritional findings/problems identified that relate to knowledge, attitudes/beliefs, physical environment, or access to food and food safety"**	NB		
Class: Knowledge and Beliefs (1)			

NUTRITION DIAGNOSIS TERMS AND DEFINITIONS

Defined as "actual knowledge and beliefs as reported, observed, or documented"			
Food and nutrition-related knowledge deficit	NB-1.1	Incomplete or inaccurate knowledge about food, nutrition or nutrition-related information and guidelines, e.g., nutrient requirements, consequences of food behaviors, life stage requirements, nutrition recommendations, diseases and conditions, physiological function, or products	123-124
Harmful beliefs/attitudes about food or nutrition-related topics USE WITH CAUTION TO BE SENSITIVE TO PATIENT CONCERNS	NB-1.2	Beliefs/attitudes and practices about food, nutrition, and nutrition-related topics that are incompatible with sound nutrition principles, nutrition care, or disease/condition	125-126
Not ready for diet/lifestyle change	NB-1.3	Lack of perceived value of nutrition-related care benefits compared to consequences or effort required to making the change; inconsistencies with other value structure/purpose; antecedent to behavior change	127-128
Self monitoring deficit	NB-1.4	Lack of data recording to track personal progress	129-130
Disordered eating pattern	NB-1.5	Beliefs, attitudes, thoughts and behaviors related to food, eating, and weight management, including classic eating disorders as well as less severe, similar conditions that negatively impact health	131-133
Limited adherence to nutrition-related recommendations	NB-1.6	Lack of nutrition-related changes as per intervention agreed upon by client or population	134-135
Undesirable food choices	NB-1.7	Food and/or beverage choices that are inconsistent with US Recommended Dietary Intake, US Dietary Guidelines, or with the My Pyramid or with targets defined in the nutrition prescription or nutrition care process	136-137
Class: Physical Activity and Function (2) ***Defined as "actual physical activity, self-care, and quality of life problems as***			

NUTRITION DIAGNOSIS TERMS AND DEFINITIONS

reported, observed, or documented"			
Physical inactivity	NB-2.1	Low level of activity/sedentary behavior to the extent that it reduces energy expenditure and impacts health	138=139
Excessive exercise	NB-2.2	An amount of exercise that exceeds that which is necessary to improve health and/or athletic performance	140-141
Inability of lack of desire to manage self care	NB-2.3	Lack of capacity or unwillingness to implement methods to support healthful food and nutrition-related behavior	142-143
Impaired ability to prepare foods/meals	NB-2.4	Cognitive or physical impairment that prevents preparation of foods/meals	144-145
Poor nutrition quality of life	NB-2.5	Diminished Nutrition Quality of Life (NQOL) scores related to food impact, self-image, psychological factors social/interpersonal factors, physical (factors), or self-efficacy	146-147
Self feeding difficulty	NB-2.6	Impaired actions to place food in mouth	148-149
Class: Food Safety and Access (3) ***Defined as "actual problems with food access or food safety"***			
Intake of unsafe food	NB-3.1	Intake of food and/or fluids intentionally or unintentionally contaminated with toxins, poisonous products, infectious agents, microbial agents, additives, allergens, and/or agents of bioterrorism	150-151
Limited access to food	NB-3.2	Diminished ability to acquire food from sources (e.g., shopping, gardening, meal delivery), due to financial constraints, physical impairment, caregiver support, or unsafe living conditions (e.g. crime hinders travel to grocery store). Limiting food intake because of concerns about weight or aging.	152-153

HYPERMETABOLISM (NI-1.1)

Definition

Resting metabolic rate (RMR) above predicted requirements due to stress, trauma, injury, sepsis, or disease. Note: RMR is the sum of metabolic processes of active cell mass related to the maintenance of normal body functions and regulatory balance during rest.

Etiology *(Cause/Contributing Risk Factors)*

Factors gathered during the nutrition assessment process that contribute to the existence or the maintenance of pathophysiological, psychosocial, situational, developmental, cultural, and/or environmental problems:

- Catabolic illness
- Infection
- Sepsis

Signs/Symptoms *(Defining Characteristics)*

A typical cluster of subjective and objective signs and symptoms gathered during the nutrition assessment process that provide evidence that a problem exists; quantify the problem and describe its severity.

Nutrition Assessment Category	Potential Indicators of this Nutrition Diagnosis (one or more must be present)
Biochemical Data	• Insulin resistance (difficult to control blood glucose)
Anthropometric Measurements	
Physical Examination Findings	• Fever • Increased heart rate • Increased respiratory rate • Measured RMR > estimated or expected RMR
Food/Nutrition History	
Client History	• Conditions associated with a diagnosis or treatment of, e.g., AIDS/HIV, burns, chronic obstructive pulmonary disease, hip/long bone fracture, infection, surgery, trauma, hyperthyroidism (pre- or untreated), some cancers (specify) • Medications associated with ↑ RMR

HYPERMETABOLISM (NI-1.1)

References:

1. Bitz C, Toubro S, Larsen TM, Harder H, Rennie KL, Jebb SA, Astrup A. Increased 24 hour energy expenditure in Type 2 diabetes mellitus. *Diabetes Care.* 2004;27:2416-2241.
2. Dickerson RN, Roth-Yousey L. Medication effects on metabolic rate; a systematic review (Part 2). *J Am Diet Assoc.* 2005;105:1002-1009.
3. Dickerson RN, Roth-Yousey L. Medication effects on metabolic rate: a systematic review (Part 1). *J Am Diet Assoc.* 2005;105:835-841.
4. Frankenfield D, Roth-Yousey L, Compher C. Comparison of predictive equations to measured resting metabolic rate in healthy nonobese and obese individuals: a systematic review. *J Am Diet Assoc.* 2005;105:775-789.

INCREASED ENERGY EXPENDITURE (NI-1.2)

Definition

Resting metabolic rate (RMR) above predicted requirements due to body composition, medication, endocrine, neurologic, or genetic change(s). Note: RMR is the sum of metabolic processes of active cell mass related to the maintenance of normal body functions and regulatory balance during rest.

Etiology (*Cause/Contributing Risk Factors*)

Factors gathered during the nutrition assessment process that contribute to the existence or the maintenance of pathophysiological, psychosocial, situational, developmental, cultural, and/or environmental problems:

- Anabolism or growth
- Voluntary or involuntary physical activity/movement

Signs/Symptoms (*Defining Characteristics*)

A typical cluster of subjective and objective signs and symptoms gathered during the nutrition assessment process that provide evidence that a problem exists; quantify the problem and describe its severity.

Nutrition Assessment Category	Potential Indicators of this Nutrition Diagnosis (one or more must be present)
Biochemical Data	
Anthropometric Measurements	• Unintentional weight loss of 10% in 6 months, 5% in 1 month • Evidence of need for accelerated or catch up growth or weight gain in children; absence of normal growth • Increased proportional lean body mass
Physical Examination Findings	• Measured RMR > estimated or expected RMR
Food/Nutrition History	• Increased physical activity, e.g., endurance athlete
Client History	• Conditions associated with a diagnosis or treatment, e.g., Parkinson's disease, cerebral palsy, Alzheimer's disease, other dementia

Reference:

1. Frankenfield D, Roth-Yousey L, Compher C. Comparison of predictive equations to measured resting metabolic rate in healthy nonobese and obese individuals: a systematic review. *J Am Diet Assoc.* 2005;105:775-789.

HYPOMETABOLISM (NI-1.3)

Definition

Resting metabolic rate (RMR) below predicted requirements due to body composition, medications, endocrine, neurologic, or genetic changes

Etiology *(Cause/Contributing Risk Factors)*

Factors gathered during the nutrition assessment process that contribute to the existence or the maintenance of pathophysiological, psychosocial, situational, developmental, cultural, and/or environmental problems:

- Loss of lean body mass, weight loss
- Medications, e.g., midazolam, propranalol, glipizide
- Endocrine changes, e.g., hypothyroidism

Signs/Symptoms *(Defining Characteristics)*

A typical cluster of subjective and objective signs and symptoms gathered during the nutrition assessment process that provide evidence that a problem exists; quantify the problem and describe its severity.

Nutrition Assessment Category	Potential Indicators of this Nutrition Diagnosis (one or more must be present)
Biochemical Data	• Increased TSH, decreased T4, T3 (hypothyroidism)
Anthropometric Data	• Decreased weight or mid-arm muscle circumference • Weight gain (e.g., hypothyroidism) • Growth stunting or failure, based on National Center for Health Statistics (NCHS) growth standards
Physical Exam Findings	• Decreased or normal adipose and somatic protein stores • Measured RMR < estimated or expected RMR
Food/Nutrition History	
Client History	• Conditions associated with a diagnosis or treatment, e.g., hypothyroidism, anorexia nervosa, malnutrition, failure to thrive, Prader-Willi syndrome, hypotonic conditions • Bradycardia, hypotension, decreased bowl motility, slow breathing rate, low body temperature (in significant weight loss) • Cold intolerance, hair loss, decreased endurance, difficulty concentrating, decreased libido, feelings of anxiety/depression

HYPOMETABOLISM (NI-1.3)

References:

1. Brozek J. Starvation and nutritional rehabilitation; a quantitative case study. *J Am Diet Assoc.* 1952;28:917-926.
2. Collins S. Using middle upper arm circumference to assess severe adult malnutrition during famine. *JAMA.* 1996;276:391-395.
3. Detzer MJ, Leitenberg H, Poehlman ET, Rosen JC, Silberg NT, Vara LS. Resting metabolic rate in women with bulimia nervosa: a cross sectional and treatment study. *Am J Clin Nutr.* 1994;60:327-332.
4. Dickerson RN, Roth-Yousey L. Medication effects on metabolic rate: a systematic review (Part 2). *J Am Diet Assoc.* 2005;105:1002-1009.
5. Dickerson RN, Roth-Yousey L. Medication effects on metabolic rate: a systematic review (Part 1). *J Am Diet Assoc.* 2005;105:835-841.
6. Frankenfield D, Roth-Yousey L, Compher C. Comparison of predictive equations to measured resting metabolic rate in healthy nonobese and obese individuals: a systematic review. *J Am Diet Assoc.* 2005;105:775-789.
7. Kerruish KP, O'Conner JO, Humphries IRJ, Kohn MR, Clarke SD, Briody JN, Thomson EJ, Wright KA, Gaskin KJ, Baur LA. Body composition in adolescents with anorexia nervosa. *Am J Clin Nutr.* 2002;75:31-37.
8. Mollinger LA, Spurr GB, el Ghatil AZ, Barboriak JS, Rooney CB, Davidoff DD. Daily energy expenditure and basil metabolic rates of patients with spinal cord injury. *Arch Phys Med Rehabil.* 1985;66:420-426.
9. Obarzanek E, Lesem MD, Jimerson DC. Resting metabolic rate of anorexia nervosa patients during weight gain. *Am J Clin Nutr.* 1994;60:666-675.
10. Pavlovic M, Zavalic M, Corovic N, Stilinovic L, Malinar M. Loss of body mass in ex prisoners of war. *Eur J Clin Nutr.* 1993;47:808-814.

INADEQUATE ENERGY INTAKE (NI-1.4)

Definition

Energy intake that is less than energy expenditure, established reference standards, or recommendations based upon physiological needs. Exception: when the goal is weight loss or during end of life care.

Etiology *(Cause/Contributing Risk Factors)*

Factors gathered during the nutrition assessment process that contribute to the existence or the maintenance of pathophysiological, psychosocial, situational, developmental, cultural, and/or environmental problems:

- Pathologic or physiologic causes that result in increased energy requirements or decreased ability to consume sufficient energy, e.g., increased nutrient needs due to prolonged catabolic illness
- Lack of access to food or artificial nutrition, e.g., economic constraints, cultural or religious practices restricting food given to elderly and/or children
- Food- and nutrition-related knowledge deficit
- Psychological causes, e.g., depression or disordered eating

Signs/Symptoms *(Defining Characteristics)*

A typical cluster of subjective and objective signs and symptoms gathered during the nutrition assessment process that provide evidence that a problem exists; quantify the problem and describe its severity.

Nutrition Assessment Category	**Potential Indicators of this Nutrition Diagnosis (one or more must be present)**
Biochemical Data	• ↓ Chol
Anthropometric Measurements	
Physical Examination Findings	• Weight loss • Poor dentition

INADEQUATE ENERGY INTAKE (NI-1.4)

Food/Nutrition History	Reports or observations of: • Insufficient energy intake from diet compared to needs based on estimated or measured resting metabolic rate • Restriction or omission of energy dense foods from diet • Food avoidance and/or lack of interest in food • Inability to independently consume foods/fluids (diminished joint mobility of wrist, hand, or digits) • Parenteral or enteral nutrition insufficient to meet needs based on estimated or measured resting metabolic rate
Client History	• Excessive consumption of alcohol or other drugs that reduce hunger

Reference:

1. National Academy of Sciences, Institute of Medicine. *Dietary Reference Intakes for Energy, Carbohydrate, Fiber, Fat, Fatty Acids, Cholesterol, Protein, and Amino Acids.* Washington, DC: National Academy Press; 2002.

EXCESSIVE ENERGY INTAKE (NI-1.5)

Definition

Caloric intake that exceeds energy expenditure, established reference standards, or recommendations based upon physiological needs. Exception: when weight gain is desired.

Etiology *(Cause/Contributing Risk Factors)*

Factors gathered during the nutrition assessment process that contribute to the existence or the maintenance of pathophysiological, psychosocial, situational, developmental, cultural, and/or environmental problems:

- Harmful beliefs/attitudes about food, nutrition, and nutrition-related topics
- Food- and nutrition-related knowledge deficit
- Lack of access to healthful food choices, e.g., food provided by caregiver
- Lack of value for behavior change, competing values
- Mental illness, depression
- Medications that increase appetite, e.g., steroids
- Overfeeding of parenteral/enteral nutrition (TPN/EN)
- Unwilling or uninterested in reducing energy intake
- Failure to adjust for lifestyle changes and decreased metabolism, e.g., aging
- Resolution of prior hypermetabolism without reduction in intake

Signs/Symptoms *(Defining Characteristics)*

A typical cluster of subjective and objective signs and symptoms gathered during the nutrition assessment process that provide evidence that a problem exists; quantify the problem and describe its severity.

EXCESSIVE ENERGY INTAKE (NI-1.5)

Nutrition Assessment Category	Potential Indicators of this Nutrition Diagnosis (one or more must be present)
Biochemical Data	• Overfeeding of TPN/EN (usually seen early after initiation of feeding): • Hyperglycemia • Hypokalemia < 3.5 mEq/L • Hypophosphatemia <1.0 mEq/L • Abnormal liver function tests
Anthropometric Measurements	• Body fat percentage > 25% for men and > 32% for women • BMI > 25 • Weight gain
Physical Exam Findings	• Increased body adiposity • Overfeeding TPN/EN: • Increased respirations
Food/Nutrition History	• Observations or reports of intake of calorically dense foods/beverages or large portions of foods/beverages • Observations, reports, or calculation of TPN/EN above estimated or measured (e.g., indirect calorimetry) caloric expenditure • Metabolic cart/indirect calorimetry measurement, e.g., respiratory quotient > 1.0
Client History	• Conditions associated with a diagnosis or treatment of, e.g., obesity, overweight, metabolic syndrome, depression, or anxiety disorder

References:

1. McClave SA, Lowen CC, Kleber MJ, McConnell JW, Jung LY, Goldsmith LJ. Clinical use of the respiratory quotient obtained from indirect calorimetry. *J Parenter Enteral Nutr.* 2003;27:21-26.
2. McClave SA, Lowen CC, Kleber MJ, Nicholson JF, Jimmerson SC, McConnell JW, Jung LY. Are patients fed appropriately according to their caloric requirements? *J Parenter Enteral Nutr.* 1998;22:375-381.
3. Overweight and Obesity: Health Consequences. www.surgeongeneral.gov/topics/obesity/calltoaction/fact_consequences.htm. Accessed August 28, 2004.

INADEQUATE ORAL FOOD/BEVERAGE INTAKE (NI-2.1)

Definition

Oral food/beverage intake that is less than established reference standards or recommendations based upon physiological needs. Exception: when the goal is weight loss or during end of life care.

Etiology *(Cause/Contributing Risk Factors)*

Factors gathered during the nutrition assessment process that contribute to the existence or the maintenance of pathophysiological, psychosocial, situational, developmental, cultural, and/or environmental problems:

- Physiologic causes, e.g., increased nutrient needs due to prolonged catabolic illness
- Lack of access to food, e.g., economic constraints, cultural or religious practices, restricting food given to elderly and/or children
- Food- and nutrition-related knowledge deficit concerning sufficient oral food/beverage intake
- Psychological causes, e.g., depression or disordered eating

Signs/Symptoms *(Defining Characteristics)*

A typical cluster of subjective and objective signs and symptoms gathered during the nutrition assessment process that provide evidence that a problem exists; quantify the problem and describe its severity.

Nutrition Assessment Category	**Potential Indicators of this Nutrition Diagnosis (one or more must be present)**
Biochemical Data	
Anthropometric Measurements	
Physical Examination Findings	• Dry skin, dry mucous membranes, poor skin turgor • Weight loss, insufficient growth velocity
Food/Nutrition History	Reports or observations of: • Insufficient intake of energy or high-quality protein from diet when compared to requirements • Economic constraints that limit food availability

INADEQUATE ORAL FOOD/BEVERAGE INTAKE (NI-2.1)

Client History	• Conditions associated with a diagnosis or treatment of catabolic illness such as AIDS, tuberculosis, anorexia nervosa, sepsis, or infection from recent surgery), depression, acute or chronic pain • Protein and/or nutrient malabsorption • Excessive consumption of alcohol or other drugs that reduce hunger • Medications that cause anorexia

References:

1. National Academy of Sciences, Institute of Medicine. *Dietary Reference Intakes for Energy, Carbohydrate, Fiber, Fat, Fatty Acids, Cholesterol, Protein, and Amino Acids*. Washington, DC: National Academy Press; 2002.
2. National Academy of Sciences, Institute of Medicine. *Dietary Reference Intakes for Water, Potassium, Sodium, Chloride, and Sulfate*. Washington, DC: National Academy Press; 2002.

EXCESSIVE ORAL FOOD/BEVERAGE INTAKE (NI-2.2)

Definition

Oral food/beverage intake that exceeds energy expenditure, established reference standards, or recommendations based upon physiological needs. Exception: when weight gain is desired.

Etiology (*Cause/Contributing Risk Factors*)

Factors gathered during the nutrition assessment process that contribute to the existence or the maintenance of pathophysiological, psychosocial, situational, developmental, cultural, and/or environmental problems:

- Harmful beliefs/attitudes about food, nutrition, and nutrition-related topics
- Food- and nutrition-related knowledge deficit
- Lack of access to healthful food choices, e.g., food provided by caregiver
- Lack of value for behavior change, competing values
- Inability to limit or refuse offered foods
- Lack of food planning, purchasing, and preparation skills
- Loss of appetite awareness
- Medications that increase appetite, e.g., steroids, antidepressants
- Unwilling or uninterested in reducing intake

Signs/Symptoms (*Defining Characteristics*)

A typical cluster of subjective and objective signs and symptoms gathered during the nutrition assessment process that provide evidence that a problem exists; quantify the problem and describe its severity.

Nutrition Assessment Category	Potential Indicators of this Nutrition Diagnosis (one or more must be present)
Biochemical Data	• Variable high blood glucose levels • Abnormal Hgb A1C
Anthropometric Measurements	• Weight gain not attributed to fluid retention or normal growth
Physical Exam Findings	• Evidence of acanthosis nigricans

EXCESSIVE ORAL FOOD/BEVERAGE INTAKE (NI-2.2)

Food/Nutrition History	Reports or observations of: • Intake of calorically dense foods/beverages (juice, soda, or alcohol) at meals and/or snacks • Intake of large portions of foods/beverages, food groups, or specific food items • Intake that exceeds estimated or measured energy needs • Highly variable daily caloric intake • Binge eating patterns • Frequent, excessive intake of fast food or restaurant food
Client History	• Conditions associated with a diagnosis or treatment, e.g., obesity, overweight, or metabolic syndrome, depression, anxiety disorder • Resting metabolic rate measurement reflecting excess intake, e.g., respiratory quotient > 1.0

References:

1. Overweight and Obesity: Health Consequences. www.surgeongeneral.gov/topics/obesity/calltoaction/fact_consequences.htm. Accessed August 28, 2004.
2. Position of the American Dietetic Association: Weight management. *J Am Diet Assoc.* 2002;102:1145-1155.
3. Position of the American Dietetic Association: Total diet approach to communicating food and nutrition information. *J Am Diet Assoc.* 2002;102:100-108.
4. Position of the American Dietetic Association: The role of dietetics professionals in health promotion and disease prevention. *J Am Diet Assoc.* 2002;102:1680-1687.

INADEQUATE INTAKE FROM ENTERAL/PARENTERAL (EN/TPN) NUTRITION INFUSION (NI-2.3)

Definition

Enteral or parenteral infusion that provides fewer calories or nutrients compared to established reference standards or recommendations based upon physiological needs. Exception: when the goal is weight loss or during end of life care.

Etiology *(Cause/Contributing Risk Factors)*

Factors gathered during the nutrition assessment process that contribute to the existence or the maintenance of pathophysiological, psychosocial, situational, developmental, cultural, and/or environmental problems:

- Altered absorption or metabolism of nutrients, e.g., medications
- Food and nutrition-related knowledge deficit (patient/client, caregiver, supplier), e.g., incorrect formula/formulation given such as wrong enteral feeding, or missing component of TPN
- Lack of, compromised, or incorrect access for delivering EN/TPN
- Increased biological demand of nutrients, e.g., accelerated growth, wound healing, chronic infection, multiple fractures
- Intolerance of EN/TPN
- Infusion volume not reached or schedule for infusion interrupted

Signs/Symptoms *(Defining Characteristics)*

A typical cluster of subjective and objective signs and symptoms gathered during the nutrition assessment process that provide evidence that a problem exists; quantify the problem and describe its severity.

Nutrition Assessment Category	Potential Indicators of this Nutrition Diagnosis (one or more must be present)

Biochemical Data	• Cholesterol < 160 mg/dL (4.16 mmol/L)
	• Vitamin/mineral abnormalities
	  • Calcium < 9.2 mg/dL (2.3 mmol/L)
	  • Vitamin K--Prolonged prothrombin time (PT), partial thromboplastin time (PTT)
	  • Copper < 70 µg/dL (11 µmol/L)
	  • Zinc < 78 µg/dL (12 µmol/L)
	  • Iron < 50 µg/dL (9 nmol/L); iron binding capacity < 250 µg/dL (44.8 µmol/L)

INADEQUATE INTAKE FROM ENTERAL/PARENTERAL (EN/TPN) NUTRITION INFUSION (NI-2.3)

Anthropometric Measurements	• Growth failure, based on National Center for Health Statistics (NCHS) growth standards and fetal growth failure • Insufficient maternal weight gain • Lack of planned weight gain • Unintentional weight loss of 5% in 1 month or 10% in 6 months (not attributed to fluid) in adults • Any weight loss in infants and children • Underweight (BMI < 18.5)
Physical Exam Findings	• Clinical evidence of vitamin/mineral deficiency (e.g., hair loss, bleeding gums, pale nail beds, neurologic changes) • Evidence of dehydration, e.g., dry mucous membranes, poor skin turgor • Loss of skin integrity or delayed wound healing • Loss of muscle mass and/or subcutaneous fat • Nausea, vomiting, diarrhea
Food/Nutrition History	Observation or reports of: • Inadequate EN/TPN volume compared to estimated or measured (indirect calorimetry) requirements • Metabolic cart/indirect calorimetry measurement, e.g., respiratory quotient < 0.7
Client History	• Conditions associated with a diagnosis or treatment of, e.g., intestinal resection, Crohn's disease, HIV/AIDS, burns, decubitus ulcers, pre-term birth, malnutrition • Feeding tube or venous access in wrong position or removed • Altered capacity for desired levels of physical activity or exercise, easy fatigue with increased activity

References:

1. McClave SA, Spain DA, Skolnick JL, Lowen CC, Kieber MJ, Wickerham PS, Vogt JR, Looney SW. Achievement of steady state optimizes results when performing indirect calorimetry. *J Parenter Enteral Nutr*. 2003;27:16-20.
2. McClave SA, Lowen CC, Kleber MJ, McConnell JW, Jung LY, Goldsmith LJ. Clinical use of the respiratory quotient obtained from indirect calorimetry. *J Parenter Enteral Nutr*. 2003;27:21-26.
3. McClave SA, Snider HL. Clinical use of gastric residual volumes as a monitor for patients on enteral tube feeding. *J Parenter Enteral Nutr*. 2002;26(Suppl):S43-48; discussion S49-S50.
4. McClave SA, DeMeo MT, DeLegge MH, DiSario JA, Heyland DK, Maloney JP, Metheny NA, Moore FA, Scolapio JS, Spain DA, Zaloga GP. North American Summit on Aspiration in the Critically Ill Patient: consensus statement. *J Parenter Enteral Nutr*. 2002;26(Suppl):S80-S85.
5. McClave SA, McClain CJ, Snider HL. Should indirect calorimetry be used as part of nutritional assessment? *J Clin Gastroenterol*. 2001;33:14-19.
6. McClave SA, Sexton LK, Spain DA, Adams JL, Owens NA, Sullins MB, Blandford BS, Snider HL. Enteral tube feeding in the intensive care unit: factors impeding adequate delivery. *Crit Care Med*. 1999;27:1252-1256.
7. McClave SA, Lowen CC, Kleber MJ, Nicholson JF, Jimmerson SC, McConnell JW, Jung LY. Are patients fed appropriately according to their caloric requirements? *J Parenter Enteral Nutr*. 1998;22:375-381.
8. Spain DA, McClave SA, Sexton LK, Adams JL, Blanford BS, Sullins ME, Owens NA, Snider HL. Infusion protocol improves delivery of enteral tube feeding in the critical care unit. *J Parenter Enteral Nutr*. 1999;23:288-292.

EXCESSIVE INTAKE FROM ENTERAL/PARENTERAL NUTRITION (NI-2.4)

Definition

Enteral or parenteral infusion that provides more calories or nutrients compared to established reference standards or recommendations based upon physiological needs.

Etiology *(Cause/Contributing Risk Factors)*

Factors gathered during the nutrition assessment process that contribute to the existence or the maintenance of pathophysiological, psychosocial, situational, developmental, cultural, and/or environmental problems:

- Physiologic causes, e.g., decreased needs related to low activity levels with critical illness or organ failure
- Food- and nutrition-related knowledge deficit on the part of the caregiver, patient/client or clinician

Signs/Symptoms *(Defining Characteristics)*

A typical cluster of subjective and objective signs and symptoms gathered during the nutrition assessment process that provide evidence that a problem exists; quantify the problem and describe its severity.

Nutrition Assessment Category	Potential Indicators of this Nutrition Diagnosis (one or more must be present)
Biochemical Data	• Elevated BUN:creatinine ratio (protein) • Hyperglycemia (carbohydrate) • Hypercapnia • Elevated liver enzymes
Anthropometric Measurements	• Weight gain in excess of lean tissue accretion
Physical Examination Findings	• Edema with excess fluid administration
Food/Nutrition History	Report or observation of: • Documented intake from enteral or parenteral nutrients that is consistently above recommended intake for carbohydrate, protein, and fat (e.g., 36 kcal/kg for well, active adults, 25 kcal/kg or as measured by indirect calorimetry for critically ill adults, 0.8 g/kg protein for well adults, 1.5 g/kg protein for critically ill adults, 4 mg/kg/minute of dextrose for critically ill adults, 1.2 g/kg lipid for adults, or 3 g/kg for children)*

* When entering weight (i.e., gram) information into the medical record, use institution or Joint Commission Accreditation of Healthcare Organizations' approved abbreviation list.

EXCESSIVE INTAKE FROM ENTERAL/PARENTERAL NUTRITION (NI-2.4)

Client History	• Use of drugs that reduce requirements or impair metabolism of energy, protein, fat or fluid. • Unrealistic expectations of weight gain or ideal weight • Receiving significant calorie intake from lipid or dextrose infusions, or peritoneal dialysis or in association with other medical treatments

References:

1. National Academy of Sciences, Institute of Medicine. *Dietary Reference Intakes for Energy, Carbohydrate, Fiber, Fat, Fatty Acids, Cholesterol, Protein, and Amino Acids.* Washington, DC: National Academy Press, 2002.
2. National Academy of Sciences, Institute of Medicine. *Dietary Reference Intakes for Water, Potassium, Sodium, Chloride, and Sulfate.* Washington, DC: National Academy Press, 2004.
3. Aarsland A, Chinkes D, Wolfe RR. Hepatic and whole-body fat synthesis in humans during carbohydrate overfeeding. *Am J Clin Nutr.* 1997;65:1774-1782.
4. McClave SA, Lowen CC, Kleber MJ, Nicholson JF, Jimmerson JC, McConnell JW, Jung LY. Are patients fed appropriately according to their caloric requirements? *J Parenter Enteral Nutr.* 1998;22:375-381.
5. McClave SA, Lowen CC, Kleber MJ, McConnell JW, Jung LY, Goldsmith LJ. Clinical use of the respiratory quotient obtained from indirect calorimetry. *J Parenter Enteral Nutr.* 2003;27:21-26.
6. Wolfe RR, O'Donnell TF, Jr., Stone MD, Richmand DA, Burke JF. Investigation of factors determining the optimal glucose infusion rate in total parenteral nutrition. *Metabolism: Clinical & Experimental.* 1980;29:892-900.

INAPPROPRIATE INFUSION OF ENTERAL OR PARENTERAL NUTRITION (NI-2.5)

Use with caution–only after discussion with other health team members

Definition

Enteral or parenteral infusion that provides either fewer or more calories and/or nutrients or is of the wrong composition or type, is not warranted because the patient/client is able to tolerate an enteral intake, or is unsafe because of the potential for sepsis or other complications

Etiology (*Cause/Contributing Risk Factors*)

Factors gathered during the nutrition assessment process that contribute to the existence or the maintenance of pathophysiological, psychosocial, situational, developmental, cultural, and/or environmental problems:

- Physiologic causes, e.g., improvement in patient/client status, allowing return to total or partial oral diet; changes in the course of disease resulting in changes in nutrient requirements
- Product or knowledge deficit on the part of the caregiver or clinician
- End of life care if patient/client or family do not desire nutrition support

Signs/Symptoms (*Defining Characteristics*)

A typical cluster of subjective and objective signs and symptoms gathered during the nutrition assessment process that provide evidence that a problem exists; quantify the problem and describe its severity.

Nutrition Assessment Category	Potential Indicators of this Nutrition Diagnosis (one or more must be present)
Biochemical Data	• Abnormal liver function tests in patient/client on long term (more than 3-6 weeks) feeding • Abnormal levels of markers specific for various nutrients, e.g., hyperphosphatemia in patient/client receiving feedings with a high phosphorus content, hypokalemia in patient/client receiving feedings with low potassium content
Anthropometric Measurements	• Weight gain in excess of lean tissue accretion • Weight loss
Physical Examination Findings	• Edema with excess fluid administration • Complications such as fatty liver in the absence of other causes • Loss of subcutaneous fat and muscle stores

INAPPROPRIATE INFUSION OF ENTERAL OR PARENTERAL NUTRITION (NI-2.5)

Food/Nutrition History	Report or observation of: • Documented intake from enteral or parenteral nutrients that is consistently above or below recommended intake for carbohydrate, protein, and/or fat — especially related to patient/client's ability to consume an oral diet that meets needs at this point in time • Documented intake of other nutrients that is consistently above or below that recommended • Nausea, vomiting, diarrhea, high gastric residual volume
Client History	• History of enteral or parenteral nutrition intolerance

References:

1. Aarsland A, Chinkes D, Wolfe RR. Hepatic and whole-body fat synthesis in humans during carbohydrate overfeeding. *Am J Clin Nutr.* 1997;65:1774-1782.
2. McClave SA, Lowen CC, Kleber MJ, Nicholson JF, Jimmerson SC, McConnell JW, Jung LY. Are patients fed appropriately according to their caloric requirements? *J Parenter Enteral Nutr.* 1998;22:375-381.
3. McClave SA, Lowen CC, Kleber MJ, McConnell JW, Jung LY, Goldsmith LJ. Clinical use of the respiratory quotient obtained from indirect calorimetry. *J Parenter Enteral Nutr.* 2003;27:21-26.
4. National Academy of Sciences, Institute of Medicine. *Dietary Reference Intakes for Energy, Carbohydrate, Fiber, Fat, Fatty Acids, Cholesterol, Protein, and Amino Acids.* Washington, DC: National Academy Press; 2002.
5. National Academy of Sciences, Institute of Medicine. *Dietary Reference Intakes for Water, Potassium, Sodium, Chloride, and Sulfate*, Washington, DC: National Academy Press; 2004.
6. National Academy of Sciences, Institute of Medicine. *Dietary Reference Intakes for Calcium, Phosphorus, Magnesium, Vitamin D, and Fluoride.* Washington, DC: National Academy Press; 1997.
7. National Academy of Sciences, Institute of Medicine. *Dietary Reference Intakes for Vitamin C, Vitamin E, Selenium, and Carotenoids.* Washington, DC: National Academy Press; 2000.
8. Wolfe RR, O'Donnell TF, Jr., Stone MD, Richmand DA, Burke JF. Investigation of factors determining the optimal glucose infusion rate in total parenteral nutrition. *Metabolism.* 1980;29:892-900.

INADEQUATE FLUID INTAKE (NI-3.1)

Definition

Lower intake of fluid-containing foods or substances compared to established reference standards or recommendations based upon physiological needs

Etiology *(Cause/Contributing Risk Factors)*

Factors gathered during the nutrition assessment process that contribute to the existence or the maintenance of pathophysiological, psychosocial, situational, developmental, cultural, and/or environmental problems:

- Physiologic causes, e.g., increased fluid needs due to climate/temperature change; increased exercise or conditions leading to increased fluid losses; fever causing increased insensible losses, decreased thirst sensation, use of drugs that reduce thirst
- Lack of access to fluid, e.g., economic constraints, cultural or religious practices, inability to access fluid independently (such as elderly or children)
- Food- and nutrition-related knowledge deficit
- Psychological causes, e.g., depression or disordered eating; dementia resulting in decreased recognition of thirst

Signs/Symptoms *(Defining Characteristics)*

A typical cluster of subjective and objective signs and symptoms gathered during the nutrition assessment process that provide evidence that a problem exists; quantify the problem and describe its severity.

Nutrition Assessment Category	Potential Indicators of this Nutrition Diagnosis (one or more must be present)
Biochemical Data	• Plasma or serum osmolality greater than 290 mOsm/kg • ↑ BUN, ↑ Na
Anthropometric Measurements	• Acute weight loss
Physical Examination Findings	• Dry skin and mucous membranes, poor skin turgor • Urine output <30 mL/hr
Food/Nutrition History	Report or observation of: • Insufficient intake of fluid when compared to requirements • Thirst • Difficulty swallowing

INADEQUATE FLUID INTAKE (NI-3.1)

Client History	• Conditions associated with a diagnosis or treatment, e.g., Alzheimer's disease or other dementia resulting in decreased recognition of thirst, diarrhea • Use of drugs that reduce thirst

References:

1. National Academy of Sciences, Institute of Medicine. *Dietary Reference Intakes for Water, Potassium, Sodium, Chloride, and Sulfate*, Washington, DC: National Academy Press; 2004.
2. Grandjean AC, Campbell, SM. *Hydration: Fluids for Life*. Monograph Series. Washington,D.C: International Life Sciences Institute North America, 2004.
3. Grandjean AC, Reimers KJ, Buyckx ME. Hydration: Issues for the 21st Century. *Nutr Rev.* 2003;61:261-271.

EXCESSIVE FLUID INTAKE (NI-3.2)

Definition

Higher intake of fluid compared to established reference standards or recommendations based upon physiological needs

Etiology (*Cause/Contributing Risk Factors*)

Factors gathered during the nutrition assessment process that contribute to the existence or the maintenance of pathophysiological, psychosocial, situational, developmental, cultural, and/or environmental problems:

- Physiologic causes, e.g., decreased fluid losses due to kidney, liver or cardiac failure; diminished water and sodium losses due to changes in exercise or climate, syndrome of inappropriate antidiuretic hormone (SIADH)
- Food- and nutrition-related knowledge deficit
- Psychological causes, e.g., depression or disordered eating

Signs/Symptoms (*Defining Characteristics*)

A typical cluster of subjective and objective signs and symptoms gathered during the nutrition assessment process that provide evidence that a problem exists; quantify the problem and describe its severity.

Nutrition Assessment Category	**Potential Indicators of this Nutrition Diagnosis (one or more must be present)**
Biochemical Data	• Lowered plasma osmolarity (270-280 mOsm/kg), only if positive fluid balance is in excess of positive salt balance • Decreased serum sodium in SIADH
Anthropometric Measurements	• Weight gain
Physical Examination Findings	• Edema in the skin of the legs, sacral area, or diffusely; weeping of fluids from lower legs • Ascites • Pulmonary edema as evidenced by shortness of breath; orthopnea; crackles or rales
Food/Nutrition History	Report or observation of: • Fluid intake in excess of recommended intake • Excessive salt intake • Inability to tolerate solid foods necessitating a liquid diet

EXCESSIVE FLUID INTAKE (NI-3.2)

Client History	• Conditions associated with a diagnosis or treatment, e.g., end stage renal disease, nephrotic syndrome, heart failure, or liver disease • Nausea, vomiting, anorexia, headache, muscle spasms, convulsions, coma related to SIADH • Shortness of breath or dyspnea with exertion or at rest • Providing medications in large amounts of fluid • Use of drugs that impair fluid excretion

References:

1. National Academy of Sciences, Institute of Medicine. *Dietary Reference Intakes for Water, Potassium, Sodium, Chloride, and Sulfate*, Washington, DC: National Academy Press; 2004.
2. Schrier R.W. ed. *Renal and Electrolyte Disorders*.6th ed. Philadelphia, Pa: Lippincott Williams and Willkins; 2002.
3. SIADH. Available at : http://ww.nlm.nih.gov/medlineplus/ency/article/000394.

INADEQUATE BIOACTIVE SUBSTANCE INTAKE (NI-4.1)

Definition

Lower intake of bioactive substances containing foods or substances compared to established reference standards or recommendations based upon physiological needs

Etiology *(Cause/Contributing Risk Factors)*

Factors gathered during the nutrition assessment process that contribute to the existence or the maintenance of pathophysiological, psychosocial, situational, developmental, cultural, and/or environmental problems:

- Food- and nutrition-related knowledge deficit
- Limited access to food-containing substance
- Altered GI function, e.g., pain or discomfort

Signs/Symptoms *(Defining Characteristics)*

A typical cluster of subjective and objective signs and symptoms gathered during the nutrition assessment process that provide evidence that a problem exists; quantify the problem and describe its severity.

Nutrition Assessment Category	**Potential Indicators of this Nutrition Diagnosis (one or more must be present)**
Biochemical Data	
Anthropometric Measurements	
Physical Exam Findings	

Food/Nutrition History	Observations or reports of:
	• Low intake of plant foods containing:
	  • Soluble fiber, e.g., psyllium (↓ total and LDL cholesterol)
	  • Soy protein (↓ total and LDL cholesterol)
	  • β-glucan, e.g., whole oat products (↓ total and LDL cholesterol)
	  • Plant sterol and stanol esters, e.g., fortified margarines (↓ total and LDL cholesterol)
	• Lack of available foods/products with bioactive substance in markets

INADEQUATE BIOACTIVE SUBSTANCE INTAKE (NI-4.1)

Client History	• Conditions associated with a diagnosis or treatment, e.g., cardiovascular disease, elevated cholesterol • Discomfort or pain associated with intake of foods rich in bioactive substances, e.g., soluble fiber, β-glucan, soy protein

Reference:

1. Position of the American Dietetic Association: Functional foods. *J Am Diet Assoc.* 2004;104:814-826.

EXCESSIVE BIOACTIVE SUBSTANCE INTAKE (NI-4.2)

Definition

Higher intake of bioactive substances other than traditional nutrients, such as functional foods, bioactive food components, dietary supplements, or food concentrates compared to established reference standards or recommendations based upon physiological needs

Etiology *(Cause/Contributing Risk Factors)*

Factors gathered during the nutrition assessment process that contribute to the existence or the maintenance of pathophysiological, psychosocial, situational, developmental, cultural, and/or environmental problems:

- Food- and nutrition-related knowledge deficit
- Contamination, misname, mislabel, misuse, recent brand change, recent dose increase, recent formulation change of substance consumed
- Frequent intake of food containing bioactive substance
- Altered GI function, e.g., pain or discomfort

Signs/Symptoms *(Defining Characteristics)*

A typical cluster of subjective and objective signs and symptoms gathered during the nutrition assessment process that provide evidence that a problem exists; quantify the problem and describe its severity.

Nutrition Assessment Category	Potential Indicators of this Nutrition Diagnosis (one or more must be present)
Biochemical Data	• Lab values indicating excessive intake of the specific substance, such as rapid drop in cholesterol from intake of stanol or sterol esters in combination with a statin drug • Increased hepatic enzyme reflecting hepatocellular damage
Anthropometric Measurements	• Weight loss as a result of malabsorption or maldigestion
Physical Exam Findings	• Constipation or diarrhea related to excessive intake • Neurologic changes, e.g., anxiety, mental status changes • Cardiovascular changes, e.g., heart rate, EKG, blood pressure

EXCESSIVE BIOACTIVE SUBSTANCE INTAKE (NI-4.2)

Food/Nutrition History	Observations or reports of: • High intake of plant foods containing: • Soy protein (↓ total and LDL cholesterol) • β-glucan, e.g., whole oat products (↓ total and LDL cholesterol) • Plant sterol and stanol esters, e.g., fortified margarines (↓ total and LDL cholesterol) or other foods based upon dietary substance, concentrate, metabolite, constituent, extract or combination • Substances which interfere with digestion or absorption of foodstuffs • Ready access to available foods/products with bioactive substance, e.g., as from dietary supplement vendors
Client History	• Conditions associated with a diagnosis or treatment, e.g., cardiovascular disease, elevated cholesterol, hypertension • Discomfort or pain associated with intake of foods rich in bioactive substances, e.g., soluble fiber, β-glucan, soy protein • Attempts to use supplements or bioactive substances for weight loss, treat constipation, prevent or cure chronic or acute disease

References:

1. National Academy of Sciences, Institute of Medicine. *Dietary Supplements: A framework for evaluating safety.* Washington, DC: National Academy Press; 2004.
2. Position of the American Dietetic Association: Functional foods. *J Am Diet Assoc.* 2004;104:814-826.

EXCESSIVE ALCOHOL INTAKE (NI-4.3)

Definition

Intake above the suggested limits for alcohol

Etiology (*Cause/Contributing Risk Factors*)

Factors gathered during the nutrition assessment process that contribute to the existence or the maintenance of pathophysiological, psychosocial, situational, developmental, cultural, and/or environmental problems.

- Harmful beliefs/attitudes about food, nutrition, and nutrition-related topics
- Food- and nutrition-related knowledge deficit
- Lack of value for behavior change, competing values
- Alcohol addiction

Signs/Symptoms (*Defining Characteristics*)

A typical cluster of subjective and objective signs and symptoms gathered during the nutrition assessment process that provide evidence that a problem exists; quantify the problem and describe its severity.

Nutrition Assessment Category	Potential Indicators of this Nutrition Diagnosis (one or more must be present)
Biochemical Data	• Elevated aspartate aminotransferase (AST), gamma-glutamyl transferase (GGT), carbohydrate-deficient transferrin, mean corpuscular volume, blood alcohol levels
Anthropometric Measurements	
Physical Exam Findings	
Food/Nutrition History	Reports or observations of: • Intake of > 2 drinks/day (men) (1 drink = 5 oz. wine, 12 oz beer, 1 oz. distilled alcohol) • Intake of > 1 drink/day (women) (1 drink = 5 oz. wine, 12 oz beer, 1 oz. distilled alcohol) • Binge drinking • Consumption of any alcohol when contraindicated

EXCESSIVE ALCOHOL INTAKE (NI-4.3)

Client History	• Conditions associated with a diagnosis or treatment, e.g., severe hypertriglyceridemia, elevated blood pressure, depression, liver disease, pancreatitis • New medical diagnosis or change in existing diagnosis or condition • History of excessive alcohol intake • Giving birth to an infant with fetal alcohol syndrome • Drinking during pregnancy despite knowledge of risk • Unexplained falls

Reference:

1. Position of the American Dietetic Association: The role of dietetics professionals in health promotion and disease prevention. *J Am Diet Assoc.* 2002;102:1680-1687.

INCREASED NUTRIENT NEEDS (SPECIFY) (NI-5.1)

Definition

Increased need for a specific nutrient compared to established reference standards or recommendations based upon physiological needs

Etiology (*Cause/Contributing Risk Factors*)

Factors gathered during the nutrition assessment process that contribute to the existence or the maintenance of pathophysiological, psychosocial, situational, developmental, cultural, and/or environmental problems:

- Altered absorption or metabolism of nutrient, e.g., from medications
- Compromise of organs related to GI function, e.g., pancreas, liver
- Decreased functional length of intestine, e.g., short bowel syndrome
- Decreased or compromised function of intestine, e.g., celiac disease, Crohn's disease
- Food- and nutrition-related knowledge deficit
- Increased demand of nutrient, e.g., accelerated growth, wound healing, chronic infection

Signs/Symptoms (*Defining Characteristics*)

A typical cluster of subjective and objective signs and symptoms gathered during the nutrition assessment process that provide evidence that a problem exists; quantify the problem and describe its severity.

Nutrition Assessment Category	Potential Indicators of this Nutrition Diagnosis (one or more must be present)
Biochemical Data	• Decreased cholesterol < 160 mg/dL, albumin, prealbumin, C-reactive protein, indicating increased stress and increased metabolic needs • Electrolyte/mineral (e.g., potassium, magnesium, phosphorus) abnormalities • Urinary or fecal losses of specific or related nutrient (e.g., fecal fat, d-xylose test) • Vitamin and/or mineral deficiency
Anthropometric Measurements	• Growth failure, based on National Center for Health Statistics (NCHS) growth standards and fetal growth failure • Unintentional weight loss of 5% in 1 month or 10% in 6 months • Underweight (BMI < 18.5)

INCREASED NUTRIENT NEEDS (SPECIFY) (NI-5.1)

Physical Examination Findings	• Clinical evidence of vitamin/mineral deficiency (e.g., hair loss, bleeding gums, pale nail beds) • Loss of skin integrity or delayed wound healing • Loss of muscle mass, subcutaneous fat
Food/Nutrition History	Observation or reports of: • Inadequate intake of foods/supplement containing needed nutrient as compared to estimated requirements • Intake of foods that do not contain sufficient quantities of available nutrient (e.g., overprocessed, overcooked, or stored improperly) • Food and nutrition-related knowledge deficit (e.g., lack of information, incorrect information or noncompliance with intake of needed nutrient)
Client History	• Fever • Conditions associated with a diagnosis or treatment, e.g., intestinal resection, Crohn's disease, HIV/AIDS, burns, pressure ulcers, pre-term birth, malnutrition • Medications affecting absorption or metabolism of needed nutrient

References:

1. Beyer P. Gastrointestinal disorders: Roles of nutrition and the dietetics practitioner. *J Am Diet Assoc.* 1998;98:272-277.
2. Position of the American Dietetic Association and Dietitians of Canada: Nutrition intervention in the care of persons with human immunodeficiency virus infection. *J Am Diet Assoc.* 2004;104:1425-1441.

EVIDENT PROTEIN-ENERGY MALNUTRITION (NI-5.2)

Definition

Inadequate intake of protein and/or energy over prolonged periods of time resulting in loss of fat stores and/or muscle wasting

Etiology *(Cause/Contributing Risk Factors)*

Factors gathered during the nutrition assessment process that contribute to the existence or the maintenance of pathophysiological, psychosocial, situational, developmental, cultural, and/or environmental problems:

- Physiologic causes, e.g., altered nutrient needs due to prolonged catabolic illness, malabsorption
- Lack of access to food, e.g., economic constraints, cultural or religious practices, restricting food given to elderly and/or children
- Food- and nutrition-related knowledge deficit, e.g., avoidance of high quality protein foods
- Psychological causes, e.g., depression or eating disorders

Signs/Symptoms *(Defining Characteristics)*

A typical cluster of subjective and objective signs and symptoms gathered during the nutrition assessment process that provide evidence that a problem exists; quantify the problem and describe its severity.

Nutrition Assessment Category	Potential Indicators of this Nutrition Diagnosis (one or more must be present)
Biochemical Data	• Normal serum albumin level (uncomplicated malnutrition) • Albumin < 3.4 mg/dL (disease/trauma-related malnutrition)
Anthropometric Measurements	• BMI < 18.5 indicates underweight • Failure to thrive, e.g. failure to attain desirable growth rates • Inadequate maternal weight gain • Weight loss of > 10% in 6 months or 5% in 1 month • Underweight with muscle wasting • Normal or slightly underweight, stunted growth in children

EVIDENT PROTEIN-ENERGY MALNUTRITION (NI-5.2)

Physical Exam Findings	• Uncomplicated malnutrition: Thin, wasted appearance; severe muscle wasting; minimal body fat; sparse, thin, dry, easily pluckable hair; dry, thin skin; obvious bony prominences, occipital wasting; lowered body temperature, blood pressure, heart rate; changes in hair or nails consistent with insufficient protein intake • Disease/trauma-related malnutrition: Thin to normal appearance, with peripheral edema, ascites or anasarca; some muscle wasting with retention of some body fat; enlarged fatty liver; dyspigmentation of hair (flag sign) and skin • Delayed wound healing
Food/Nutrition History	Reports or observations of: • Insufficient energy intake from diet compared to estimated or measured RMR • Insufficient intake of high-quality protein when compared to requirements • Food avoidance and/or lack of interest in food
Client History	• Chronic or acute disease or trauma, geographic location and socioeconomic status associated with altered nutrient intake of indigenous phenomenon • Severe protein and/or nutrient malabsorption (e.g. extensive bowel resection) • Excessive consumption of alcohol or other drugs that reduce hunger

References:

1. Wellcome Trust Working Party. Classification of infantile malnutrition. *Lancet.* 1970;2:302-303.
2. Seres DS, Resurrection, LB. Kwashiorkor: Dysmetabolism versus malnutrition. *Nutr Clin Pract.* 2003;18:297-301.
3. Jelliffe DB, Jelliffe EF. Causation of kwashiorkor: Toward a multifactoral consensus. *Pediatrics* 1992:90:110-113.
4. Centers for Disease Control and Prevention Web site. Available at: http://www.cdc.gov/nccdphp/dnpa/bmi/bmi-adult.htm. Accessed October 5, 2004.
5. Fuhrman MP, Charney P, Mueller CM. Hepatic proteins and nutrition assessment. *J Am Diet Assoc.* 2004;104:1258-1264.
6. U.S. Department of Health and Human Services. *The International Classification of Diseases,* 9th Revision, 4th ed. Washington DC: USDHSS Publication No. (PHS) 91-1260; 1991.

INADEQUATE PROTEIN-ENERGY INTAKE (NI-5.3)

Definition

Inadequate intake of protein and/or energy compared to established reference standards or recommendations based upon physiological needs of short or recent duration

Etiology *(Cause/Contributing Risk Factors)*

Factors gathered during the nutrition assessment process that contribute to the existence or the maintenance of pathophysiological, psychosocial, situational, developmental, cultural, and/or environmental problems.

- Short-term physiologic causes, e.g., increased nutrient needs due to catabolic illness, malabsorption
- Recent lack of access to food, e.g., economic constraints, cultural or religious practices, restricting food given or food selected
- Food- and nutrition-related knowledge deficit, e.g., avoidance of all fats for new dieting pattern
- Recent onset of psychological causes, e.g., depression or eating disorders

Signs/Symptoms *(Defining Characteristics)*

A typical cluster of subjective and objective signs and symptoms gathered during the nutrition assessment process that provide evidence that a problem exists; quantify the problem and describe its severity.

Nutrition Assessment Category	Potential Indicators of this Nutrition Diagnosis (one or more must be present)
Biochemical Data	• Normal albumin (in the setting of normal liver function despite decrease protein-energy intake)
Anthropometric Measurements	• Inadequate maternal weight gain (mild but not severe) • Weight loss of 5-7% over past 3 months in adults, any weight loss in children • Normal or slightly underweight • Growth failure in children
Physical Exam Findings	• Slow wound healing in pressure ulcer or surgical patient/client

INADEQUATE PROTEIN-ENERGY INTAKE (NI-5.3)

Food/Nutrition History	Reports or observations of: • Insufficient energy intake from diet compared to estimated or measured resting metabolic rate (RMR) or recommended levels • Restriction or omission of food groups such as dairy or meat group foods (protein); bread or milk group foods (energy) • Recent food avoidance and/or lack of interest in food • Lack of ability to prepare meals
Client History	• Conditions associated with a diagnosis or treatment of mild protein-energy malnutrition, recent illness, e.g. pulmonary or cardiac failure, flu, infection, surgery • Nutrient malabsorption (e.g. bariatric surgery, diarrhea, steatorrhea) • Excessive consumption of alcohol or other drugs that reduce hunger • Patient/client reports of hunger in the face of inadequate access to food supply • Patient/client reports lack of ability to prepare meals • Patient/client reports lack of funds for purchase of appropriate foods

References:

1. Centers for Disease Control and Prevention Web site. Available at: http://www.cdc.gov/nccdphp/dnpa/bmi/bmi-adult.htm. Accessed October 5, 2004.
2. Fuhrman MP, Charney P, Mueller CM. Hepatic proteins and nutrition assessment. *J Am Diet Assoc.* 2004;104:1258-1264.
3. U.S. Department of Health and Human Services. *The International Classification of Diseases,* 9th Revision, 4th ed. Washington DC: USDHSS Publication No. (PHS) 91-1260; 1991.

DECREASED NUTRIENT NEEDS (SPECIFY) (NI-5.4)

Definition

Decreased need for a specific nutrient compared to established reference standards or recommendations based upon physiological needs

Etiology *(Cause/Contributing Risk Factors)*

Factors gathered during the nutrition assessment process that contribute to the existence or the maintenance of pathophysiological, psychosocial, situational, developmental, cultural, and/or environmental problems:

- Renal dysfunction
- Liver dysfunction
- Altered cholesterol metabolism/regulation
- Heart failure
- Food intolerances, e.g., irritable bowel syndrome

Signs/Symptoms *(Defining Characteristics)*

A typical cluster of subjective and objective signs and symptoms gathered during the nutrition assessment process that provide evidence that a problem exists; quantify the problem and describe its severity.

Nutrition Assessment Category	Potential Indicators of this Nutrition Diagnosis (one or more must be present)
Biochemical Data	• Cholesterol > 200 mg/dL (5.2 mmol/L), LDL cholesterol > 100 mg/dL (2.59 mmol/L), HDL cholesterol < 40 mg/dL (1.036 mmol/L), triglycerides > 150 mg/dL (1.695 mmol/L) • Phosphorus > 5.5 mg/dL (1.78 mmol/L) • Glomerular filtration rate (GFR) < 90 mL/min/1.73 m^2 • Elevated BUN, Cr, potassium • Liver function tests indicating severe liver disease
Anthropometric Measurements	
Physical Exam Findings	• Edema/fluid retention • Interdialytic weight gain greater than expected

DECREASED NUTRIENT NEEDS (SPECIFY) (NI-5.4)

Food/Nutrition History	Reports or observations of: • Intake higher than recommended for fat, phosphorus, sodium, protein, fiber
Client History	• Conditions associated with a diagnosis or treatment that require a specific type and/or amount of nutrient, e.g., cardiovascular disease (fat), early renal disease (protein, phosphorus), ESRD (phosphorus, sodium, potassium, fluid), advanced liver disease (protein), heart failure (sodium, fluid), irritable bowel disease/Crohn's disease flare up (fiber) • Diagnosis of hypertension, confusion related to liver disease

References:

1. Aparicio M, Chauveau P, Combe C. Low protein diets and outcomes of renal patients. *J Nephrol.* 2001;14:433-439.
2. Beto JA, Bansal VK. Medical nutrition therapy in chronic kidney failure: Integrating clinical practice guidelines. *J Am Diet Assoc.* 2004;104:404-409.
3. Cupisti A, Morelli E, D'Alessandro C, Lupetti S, Barsotti G. Phosphate control in chronic uremia: don't forget diet. *J Nephrol.* 2003;16:29-33.
4. Durose CL, Holdsworth M, Watson V, Przygrodzka F. Knowledge of dietary restrictions and the medical consequences of noncompliance by patients on hemodialysis are not predictive of dietary compliance. *J Am Diet Assoc.* 2004;104:35-41.
5. Floch MH, Narayan R. Diet in the irritable bowel syndrome. *Clin Gastroenterol.* 2002;35:S45-S52.
6. Kato J, Kobune M, Nakamura T, Kurojwa G, Takada K, Takimoto R, Sato Y, Fujikawa K, Takahashi M, Takayama T, Ikeda T, Niitsu Y. Normalization of elevated hepatic 8-hydroxy-2'-deoxyguanosine levels in chronic hepatitis C patients by phlebotomy and low iron diet. *Cancer Res.* 2001;61:8697-8702.
7. Lee SH, Molassiotis A. Dietary and fluid compliance in Chinese hemodialysis patients. *Int J Nurs Stud.* 2002;39:695-704.
8. Poduval RD, Wolgemuth C, Ferrell J, Hammes MS. Hyperphosphatemia in dialysis patients: is there a role for focused counseling? *J Ren Nutr.* 2003;13:219-223.
9. Tandon N, Thakur V, Guptan RK, Sarin SK. Beneficial influence of an indigenous low-iron diet on serum indicators of iron status in patients with chronic liver disease. *Br J Nutr.* 2000;83:235-239.
10. Zrinyi M, Juhasz M, Balla J, Katona E, Ben T, Kakuk G, Pall D. Dietary self-efficacy: determinant of compliance behaviours and biochemical outcomes in haemodialysis patients. *Nephrol Dial Transplant.* 2003;19:1869-1873.

IMBALANCE OF NUTRIENTS (NI-5.5)

Definition

An undesirable combination of ingested nutrients, such that the amount of one nutrient ingested interferes with or alters absorption and/or utilization of another nutrient

Etiology *(Cause/Contributing Risk Factors)*

Factors gathered during the nutrition assessment process that contribute to the existence or the maintenance of pathophysiological, psychosocial, situational, developmental, cultural, and/or environmental problems:

- Consumption of high dose nutrient supplements
- Food- and nutrition-related knowledge deficit
- Harmful beliefs/attitudes about food, nutrition, and nutrition-related information
- Food faddism

Signs/Symptoms *(Defining Characteristics)*

A typical cluster of subjective and objective signs and symptoms gathered during the nutrition assessment process that provide evidence that a problem exists; quantify the problem and describe its severity.

Nutrition Assessment Category	Potential Indicators of this Nutrition Diagnosis (one or more must be present)
Biochemical Data	
Anthropometric Data	
Physical Exam Findings	
Food/Nutrition History	Reports or observations of: • High intake of iron supplements (↓ zinc absorption) • High intake of zinc supplements (↓ copper status) • High intake of manganese (↓ iron status)
Client History	• Diarrhea or constipation (iron supplements) • Epigastric pain, nausea, vomiting, diarrhea (zinc supplements) • Contributes to the development of anemia (manganese supplements)

IMBALANCE OF NUTRIENTS (NI-5.5)

References:

1. National Academy of Sciences, Institute of Medicine. *Dietary Reference Intakes for Vitamin A, Vitamin K, Arsenic, Boron, Chromium, Copper, Iodine, Iron, Manganese, Molybdenum, Nickel, Silicon, Vanadium, Zinc*. Washington, DC: National Academy Press; 2001.
2. National Academy of Sciences, Institute of Medicine. *Dietary Reference Intakes for Calcium, Phosphorus, Magnesium, Vitamin D, and Fluoride*. Washington, DC: National Academy Press; 1997

INADEQUATE FAT INTAKE (NI-51.1)

Definition

Lower fat intake compared to established reference standards or recommendations based upon physiological needs. Exception: when the goal is weight loss or during end of life care.

Etiology *(Cause/Contributing Risk Factors)*

Factors gathered during the nutrition assessment process that contribute to the existence or the maintenance of pathophysiological, psychosocial, situational, developmental, cultural, and/or environmental problems:

- Inappropriate food choices, e.g., economic constraints, cultural or religious practices, restricting food given to elderly and/or children, specific food choices
- Food- and nutrition-related knowledge deficit, e.g,. prolonged adherence to a very low fat diet
- Psychological causes, e.g., depression or disordered eating

Signs/Symptoms *(Defining Characteristics)*

A typical cluster of subjective and objective signs and symptoms gathered during the nutrition assessment process that provide evidence that a problem exists; quantify the problem and describe its severity.

Nutrition Assessment Category	Potential Indicators of this Nutrition Diagnosis (one or more must be present)
Biochemical Data	• Triene:tetraene ratio >0.2
Anthropometric Measurements	• Weight loss if insufficient calories consumed
Physical Examination Findings	• Rough, scaly skin that becomes dermatitis with essential fatty acid deficiency
Food/Nutrition History	Report or observation of • Intake of essential fatty acid containing foods consistently providing less than 10% of calories
Client History	• Conditions associated with a diagnosis or treatment, e.g., prolonged catabolic illness (e.g., AIDS, tuberculosis, anorexia nervosa, sepsis or severe infection from recent surgery) • Severe fat malabsorption with bowel resection, pancreatic insufficiency, or hepatic disease accompanied by steatorrhea

References:

1. National Academy of Sciences, Institute of Medicine. *Dietary Reference Intakes for Energy, Carbohydrate, Fiber, Fat, Fatty Acids, Cholesterol, Protein, and Amino Acids.* Washington, DC: National Academy Press; 2002.

EXCESSIVE FAT INTAKE (NI-51.2)

Definition

Higher fat intake compared to established reference standards or recommendations based upon physiological needs

Etiology (*Cause/Contributing Risk Factors*)

Factors gathered during the nutrition assessment process that contribute to the existence or the maintenance of pathophysiological, psychosocial, situational, developmental, cultural, and/or environmental problems:

- Food- and nutrition-related knowledge deficit
- Harmful beliefs/attitudes about food, nutrition, and nutrition-related topics
- Lack of access to healthful food choices, e.g., food provided by caregiver
- Changes in taste and appetite or preference
- Lack of value for behavior change; competing values

Signs/Symptoms (*Defining Characteristics*)

A typical cluster of subjective and objective signs and symptoms gathered during the nutrition assessment process that provide evidence that a problem exists; quantify the problem and describe its severity.

Nutrition Assessment Category	Potential Indicators of this Nutrition Diagnosis (one or more must be present)
Biochemical Data	• Cholesterol >200 mg/dL (5.2 mmol/L), LDL cholesterol > 100 mg/dL (2.59 mmol/L), HDL cholesterol < 40 mg/dL (1.036 mmol/L), triglycerides > 150 mg/dL (1.695 mmol/L) • Elevated serum amylase and/or lipase • Elevated liver function tests and/or total bilirubin • Triene:tetraene ratio > 0.4 • Fecal fat > 7g/ 24 hours
Anthropometric Measurements	
Physical Exam Findings	• Evidence of xanthomas • Evidence of skin lesions

EXCESSIVE FAT INTAKE (NI-51.2)

Food/Nutrition History	Reports or observations of: • Frequent or large portions of high-fat foods • Frequent food preparation with added fat • Frequent consumption of high-risk lipids (i.e., saturated fat, *trans* fat, cholesterol) • Report of foods containing fat above diet prescription • Inadequate intake of essential lipids
Client History	• Conditions associated with a diagnosis or treatment, e.g., hyperlipidemia, cystic fibrosis, angina, artherosclerosis, pancreatic, liver, and biliary diseases; post-transplantation • Medication, e.g., pancreatic enzymes, cholesterol, or other lipid-lowering medications • Diarrhea, cramping, steatorrhea, epigastric pain • Family history of hyperlipidemia, atherosclerosis, or pancreatitis.

References:

1. National Academy of Sciences, Institute of Medicine. *Dietary Reference Intakes for Energy, Carbohydrate, Fiber, Fat, Fatty Acids, Cholesterol, Protein, and Amino Acids.* Washington, DC: National Academy Press; 2002.
2. Position of the American Dietetic Association: Weight management. *J Am Diet Assoc.* 2002;102:1145-1155.
3. Position of the American Dietetic Association: Total diet approach to communicating food and nutrition information. *J Am Diet Assoc.* 2002;102:100-108.
4. Position of the American Dietetic Association: The role of dietetics professionals in health promotion and disease prevention. *J Am Diet Assoc.* 2002;102:1680-1687.

INAPPROPRIATE INTAKE OF FOOD FATS (NI-51.3)

Definition

Intake of wrong type or quality of food fats compared to established reference standards or recommendations based upon physiological needs

Etiology *(Cause/Contributing Risk Factors)*

Factors gathered during the nutrition assessment process that contribute to the existence or the maintenance of pathophysiological, psychosocial, situational, developmental, cultural, and/or environmental problems:

- Food- and nutrition-related knowledge deficit
- Harmful beliefs/attitudes about food, nutrition, and nutrition-related topics
- Lack of access to healthful food choices, e.g., food provided by caregiver, pediatrics, homeless
- Changes in taste and appetite or preference
- Lack of value for behavior change; competing values

Signs/Symptoms *(Defining Characteristics)*

A typical cluster of subjective and objective signs and symptoms gathered during the nutrition assessment process that provide evidence that a problem exists; quantify the problem and describe its severity.

Nutrition Assessment Category	Potential Indicators of this Nutrition Diagnosis (one or more must be present)
Biochemical Data	• Cholesterol >200 mg/dL (5.2 mmol/L), LDL cholesterol > 100 mg/dL (2.59 mmol/L), HDL cholesterol < 40 mg/dL (1.036 mmol/L), triglycerides > 150 mg/dL (1.695 mmol/L) • Elevated serum amylase and/or lipase • Elevated liver function tests, total bilirubin, and C-reactive protein
Anthropometric Measurements	
Physical Exam Findings	• Evidence of xanthomas • Evidence of skin lesions

INAPPROPRIATE INTAKE OF FOOD FATS (NI-51.3)

Food/Nutrition History	Reports or observations of: • Frequent food preparation with added fat that is not of desired type for condition • Frequent consumption of fats that are undesirable for condition (i.e., saturated fat, *trans* fat, cholesterol, omega-6 fatty acids) • Inadequate intake of monounsaturated, polyunsaturated, or omega-3 fatty acids
Client History	• Conditions associated with a diagnosis or treatment of diabetes, cardiac diseases, obesity, liver or biliary disorders • Diarrhea, cramping, steatorrhea, epigastric pain • Family history of diabetes-related heart disease, hyperlipidemia, atherosclerosis, or pancreatitis • Client desires to implement a Mediterranean-type diet

References:

1. de Lorgeril M, Salen P, Martin JL, Monjaud I, Delaye J, Mamelle N. Mediterranean diet, traditional risk factors, and the rate of cardiovascular complications after myocardial infarction. Final report of the Lyon Diet Heart Study. *Circulation.* 1999;99:779-785.
2. Franz MJ, Bantle JP, Beebe CA, Brunzell JD, Chiasson J-L, Garg A, Holzmeister LA, Hoogwerf B, Mayer-Davis E, Mooradian AD, Purnell JQ, Wheeler M: Technical review. Evidence-based nutrition principles and recommendations for the treatment and prevention of diabetes and related complications. *Diabetes Care.* 2002;202:148-198.
3. Knoops KTB, de Grott LCPGM, Kromhout D, Perrin A-E, Varela MV, Menotti A, van Staveren WA. Mediterranean diet, lifestyle factors, and 10-year mortality in elderly European men and women. *JAMA.* 2004;292:1433-1439,
4. Kris-Etherton PM, Harris WS, Appel LJ, for the Nutrition Committee. AHA scientific statement. Fish consumption, fish oil, omega-3 fatty acids, and cardiovascular disease. *Circulation.* 2002;106:2747-2757.
5. Panagiotakos DB, Pitsavos C, Polychronopoulos E, Chrysohoou C, Zampelas A, Trichopoulou A. Can a Mediterranean diet moderate the development and clinical progression of coronary heart disease? A systematic review. *Med Sci Monit.* 2004;10:RA193-RA198.
6. Position of the American Dietetic Association: Weight management. *J Am Diet Assoc.* 2002;102:1145-1155.
7. Position of the American Dietetic Association: Total diet approach to communicating food and nutrition information. *J Am Diet Assoc.* 2002;102:100-108.
8. Position of the American Dietetic Association: The role of dietetics professionals in health promotion and disease prevention. *J Am Diet Assoc.* 2002;102:1680-1687.
9. Zhao G, Etherton TD, Martin KR, West SG, Gilles PJ, Kris-Etherton PM. Dietary alpha-linolenic acid reduces inflammatory and lipid cardiovascular risk factors in hypercholesterolemic men and women. *J Nutr.* 2004;134:2991-2997.

INADEQUATE PROTEIN INTAKE (NI-52.1)

Definition

Lower intake of protein-containing foods or substances compared to established reference standards or recommendations based upon physiological needs

Etiology *(Cause/Contributing Risk Factors)*

Factors gathered during the nutrition assessment process that contribute to the existence or the maintenance of pathophysiological, psychosocial, situational, developmental, cultural, and/or environmental problems:

- Physiologic causes, e.g., increased nutrient needs due to prolonged catabolic illness, malabsorption, age or condition
- Lack of access to food, e.g., economic constraints, cultural or religious practices, restricting food given to elderly and/or children
- Food- and nutrition-related knowledge deficit
- Psychological causes, e.g., depression or disordered eating

Signs/Symptoms *(Defining Characteristics)*

A typical cluster of subjective and objective signs and symptoms gathered during the nutrition assessment process that provide evidence that a problem exists; quantify the problem and describe its severity.

Nutrition Assessment Category	Potential Indicators of this Nutrition Diagnosis (one or more must be present)
Biochemical Data	
Anthropometric Measurements	
Physical Examination Findings	
Diet History	Report or observation of • Insufficient intake of protein to meet requirements • Cultural or religious practices that limit protein intake • Economic constraints that limit food availability • Prolonged adherence to a very low-protein weight loss diet
Client History	• Conditions associated with a diagnosis or treatment, e.g., severe protein malabsorption such as bowel resection

Reference:

1. National Academy of Sciences, Institute of Medicine. *Dietary Reference Intakes for Energy, Carbohydrate, Fiber, Fat, Fatty Acids, Cholesterol, Protein, and Amino Acids.* Washington, DC: National Academy Press; 2002.

EXCESSIVE PROTEIN INTAKE (NI-52.2)

Definition

Intake above the recommended level of protein compared to established reference standards or recommendations based upon physiological needs

Etiology *(Cause/Contributing Risk Factors)*

Factors gathered during the nutrition assessment process that contribute to the existence or the maintenance of pathophysiological, psychosocial, situational, developmental, cultural, and/or environmental problems:

- Liver dysfunction
- Renal dysfunction
- Harmful beliefs/attitudes about food, nutrition and nutrition-related topics
- Lack of access to specialized protein products
- Metabolic abnormality
- Food faddism

Signs/Symptoms *(Defining Characteristics)*

A typical cluster of subjective and objective signs and symptoms gathered during the nutrition assessment process that provide evidence that a problem exists; quantify the problem and describe its severity.

Nutrition Assessment Category	Potential Indicators of this Nutrition Diagnosis (one or more must be present)
Biochemical Data	• Altered laboratory values e.g. ↑ BUN, ↓ glomerular filtration rate (altered renal status)
Anthropometric Measurements	• Growth stunting or failure based on National Center for Health Sstatistics growth charts (metabolic disorders)
Physical Exam Findings	
Food/Nutrition History	Reports or observations of: • Higher than recommended total protein intake, e.g., early renal disease, advanced liver disease with confusion • Inappropriate supplementation
Client History	• Conditions associated with a diagnosis or treatment, e.g., early renal disease or advanced liver disease with confusion

EXCESSIVE PROTEIN INTAKE (NI-52.2)

References:

1. Position of the American Dietetic Association: Food and nutrition misinformation. *J Am Diet Assoc.* 2002;102:260-266.
2. Beto JA, Bansal VK. Medical nutrition therapy in chronic kidney failure: Integrating clinical practice guidelines. *J Am Diet Assoc.* 2004;104:404-409.
3. Brandle E, Sieberth HG, Hautmann RE. Effect of chronic dietary protein intake on the renal function in healthy subjects. *Eur J Clin Nutr.* 1996;50:734-740.
4. Frassetto LA, Todd KM, Morris RC Jr, Sebastian A. Estimation of net endogenous noncarbonic acid production in humans from diet, potassium and protein contents. *Am J Clin Nutr.* 1998;68:576-583.
5. Friedman N, ed. *Absorption and Utilization of Amino Acids, Vol. I.* Boca Raton, Fla. CRC Press; 1989:229-242.
6. Hoogeveen EK, Kostense PJ, Jager A, Heine RJ, Jakobs C, Bouter LM, Donker AJ, Stehower CD. Serum homocysteine level and protein intake are related to risk of microalbuminuria: the Hoorn study. *Kidney Int.* 1998;54:203-209.
7. Rudman D, DiFulco TJ, Galambos JT, Smith RB 3rd, Salam AA, Warren WD. Maximum rate of excretion and synthesis of urea in normal and cirrhotic subjects. *J Clin Invest.* 1973;52:2241-2249.

INAPPROPRIATE INTAKE OF AMINO ACIDS (SPECIFY) (NI-52.3)

Definition

Intake that is more or less than recommended level and/or type of amino acids compared to established reference standards or recommendations based upon physiological needs

Etiology *(Cause/Contributing Risk Factors)*

Factors gathered during the nutrition assessment process that contribute to the existence or the maintenance of pathophysiological, psychosocial, situational, developmental, cultural, and/or environmental problems:

- Liver dysfunction
- Renal dysfunction
- Harmful beliefs/attitudes about food, nutrition- and nutrition-related topics
- Misused specialized protein products
- Metabolic abnormality
- Food faddism
- Inborn errors of metabolism

Signs/Symptoms *(Defining Characteristics)*

A typical cluster of subjective and objective signs and symptoms gathered during the nutrition assessment process that provide evidence that a problem exists; quantify the problem and describe its severity.

Nutrition Assessment Category	Potential Indicators of this Nutrition Diagnosis (one or more must be present)
Biochemical Data	• Altered laboratory values, e.g., ↑ BUN, ↓ glomerular filtration rate (altered renal status); increased urinary 3-methyl-histidine • Elevated specific amino acids (inborn errors of metabolism) • Uremia, azotemia (renal patients) • Elevated homocysteine or ammonia
Anthropometric Measurements	
Physical Exam Findings	• Physical or neurological changes (inborn errors of metabolism)

INAPPROPRIATE INTAKE OF AMINO ACIDS (SPECIFY) (NI-52.3)

Food/Nutrition History	Reports or observations of: • Higher than recommended amino acid intake, e.g., early renal disease, advanced liver disease, inborn error of metabolism • Higher than recommended type of amino acids for prescribed EN or TPN therapy • Inappropriate supplementation, as for athletes • Higher than recommended type of protein, e.g., excess phenylalanine intake
Client History	• Conditions associated with a diagnosis or treatment of illness that requires EN or TPN therapy • History of use of amino acids or protein powders for athletic enhancement • History of inborn error of metabolism

References:

1. Beto JA, Bansal VK. Medical nutrition therapy in chronic kidney failure: Integrating clinical practice guidelines. *J Am Diet Assoc.* 2004;104:404-409.
2. Brandle E, Sieberth HG, Hautmann RE. Effect of chronic dietary protein intake on the renal function in healthy subjects. *Eur J Clin Nutr.* 1996;50:734-740.
3. Cohn RM, Roth KS. Hyperammonia, bane of the brain. *Clin Pediatr.* 2004;43:683-689.
4. Frassetto LA, Todd KM, Morris RC Jr, Sebastian A. Estimation of net endogenous noncarbonic acid production in humans from diet, potassium and protein contents. *Am J Clin Nutr.* 1998;68:576-583.
5. Friedman N, ed. *Absorption and Utilization of Amino Acids, Vol. I.* Boca Raton, Fla:CRC Press; 1989:229-242.
6. Hoogeveen EK, Kostense PJ, Jager A, Heine RJ, Jakobs C, Bouter LM, Donker AJ, Stehower CD. Serum homocysteine level and protein intake are related to risk of microalbuminuria: the Hoorn study. *Kidney Int.* 1998;54:203-209.
7. Position of the American Dietetic Association: Food and nutrition misinformation. *J Am Diet Assoc.* 2002;102:260-266.
8. Rudman D, DiFulco TJ, Galambos JT, Smith RB 3rd, Salam AA, Warren WD. Maximum rate of excretion and synthesis of urea in normal and cirrhotic subjects. *J Clin Invest.* 1973;52:2241-2249.

INADEQUATE CARBOHYDRATE INTAKE (NI-53.1)

Definition

Lower intake of carbohydrate-containing foods or substances compared to established reference standards or recommendations based upon physiological needs

Etiology (*Cause/Contributing Risk Factors*)

Factors gathered during the nutrition assessment process that contribute to the existence or the maintenance of pathophysiological, psychosocial, situational, developmental, cultural, and/or environmental problems:

- Physiologic causes, e.g., increased energy needs due to increased activity level or metabolic change, malabsorption
- Lack of access to food, e.g., economic constraints, cultural or religious practices, restricting food given to elderly and/or children
- Food- and nutrition-related knowledge deficit
- Psychological causes, e.g., depression or disordered eating

Signs/Symptoms (*Defining Characteristics*)

A typical cluster of subjective and objective signs and symptoms gathered during the nutrition assessment process that provide evidence that a problem exists; quantify the problem and describe its severity.

Nutrition Assessment Category	**Potential Indicators of this Nutrition Diagnosis (one or more must be present)**
Biochemical Data	
Anthropometric Measurements	
Physical Examination Findings	• Ketone smell on breath
Diet History	Report or observation of: • Carbohydrate intake below recommended amounts • Inability to independently consume foods/fluids, e.g., diminished mobility in hand, wrist, or digits
Client History	• Conditions associated with a diagnosis or treatment, e.g., pancreatic insufficiency, hepatic disease, celiac disease, seizure disorder, carbohydrate malabsorption, or low-carbohydrate diets

Reference:

1. National Academy of Sciences, Institute of Medicine. *Dietary Reference Intakes for Energy, Carbohydrate, Fiber, Fat, Fatty Acids, Cholesterol, Protein, and Amino Acids*. Washington, DC: National Academy Press; 2002.

EXCESSIVE CARBOHYDRATE INTAKE (NI-53.2)

Definition

Intake above the recommended level and type of carbohydrate compared to established reference standards or recommendations based upon physiological needs

Etiology *(Cause/Contributing Risk Factors)*

Factors gathered during the nutrition assessment process that contribute to the existence or the maintenance of pathophysiological, psychosocial, situational, developmental, cultural, and/or environmental problems:

- Physiologic causes requiring modified carbohydrate intake, e.g., diabetes mellitus, lactase deficiency, sucrase-isomaltase deficiency, aldolase-B deficiency
- Cultural or religious practices that interfere with the ability to reduce carbohydrate intake
- Food- and nutrition-related knowledge deficit, e.g., inability to access sufficient information concerning appropriate carbohydrate intake
- Food and nutrition compliance limitations, e.g., lack of willingness or failure to modify carbohydrate intake in response to recommendations from a dietitian or physician
- Psychological causes, e.g., depression or disordered eating

Signs/Symptoms *(Defining Characteristics)*

A typical cluster of subjective and objective signs and symptoms gathered during the nutrition assessment process that provide evidence that a problem exists; quantify the problem and describe its severity.

Nutrition Assessment Category	Potential Indicators of this Nutrition Diagnosis (one or more must be present)
Biochemical Data	• Hyperglycemia (fasting blood sugar > 126 mg/dL) • Hemoglobin A1C > 6% • Abnormal oral glucose tolerance test (2-hour postload glucose > 200 mg/dL)
Anthropometric Measurements	
Physical Examination Findings	• Dental caries • Diarrhea in response to carbohydrate feeding

EXCESSIVE CARBOHYDRATE INTAKE (NI-53.2)

Food/Nutrition History	Reports or observations of: • Cultural or religious practices that do not support modification of dietary carbohydrate intake • Economic constraints that limit availability of appropriate foods • Carbohydrate intake that is consistently above recommended amounts
Client History	• Conditions associated with a diagnosis or treatment, e.g., diabetes mellitus, inborn errors of carbohydrate metabolism, lactase deficiency, severe infection, sepsis, or obesity • Chronic use of medications that cause hyperglycemia, e.g., steroids • Pancreatic insufficiency resulting in reduced insulin production

References:

1. Bowman BA, Russell RM. *Present Knowledge in Nutrition.* 8th ed. Washington, DC: ILSI Press; 2001.
2. Clement S, Braithwaite SS, Magee MF, Ahmann A, Smith EP, Schafer RG, Hirsch IB, American Diabetes Association Diabetes in Hospitals Writing Committee. Management of diabetes in hospitals. *Diabetes Care*. 2004;27:553-592.
3. National Academy of Sciences, Institute of Medicine. *Dietary Reference Intakes for Energy, Carbohydrate, Fiber, Fat, Fatty Acids, Cholesterol, Protein, and Amino Acids.* Washington, DC: National Academy Press; 2002.
4. The Expert Committee on the Diagnosis and Classification of Diabetes Mellitus. Diagnosis and classification of diabetes mellitus. *Diabetes Care*. 2004;27:S5-S10.

INAPPROPRIATE INTAKE OF TYPES OF CARBOHYDRATES (SPECIFY) (NI-53.3)

Definition

Intake or the type or amount of carbohydrate that is above or below the established reference standards or recommendations based upon physiological needs

Etiology *(Cause/Contributing Risk Factors)*

Factors gathered during the nutrition assessment process that contribute to the existence or the maintenance of pathophysiological, psychosocial, situational, developmental, cultural, and/or environmental problems:

- Physiologic causes requiring careful use of modified carbohydrate, e.g., diabetes mellitus, metabolic syndrome, hypoglycemia, celiac disease, allergies, obesity
- Cultural or religious practices that interfere with the ability to regulate types of carbohydrate consumed
- Food- and nutrition-related knowledge deficit, e.g., inability to access sufficient information concerning more appropriate carbohydrate types and/or amounts
- Food and nutrition compliance limitations, e.g., lack of willingness or failure to modify carbohydrate intake in response to recommendations from a dietitian, physician, or caregiver
- Psychological causes, e.g., depression or disordered eating

Signs/Symptoms *(Defining Characteristics)*

A typical cluster of subjective and objective signs and symptoms gathered during the nutrition assessment process that provide evidence that a problem exists; quantify the problem and describe its severity.

Nutrition Assessment Category	Potential Indicators of this Nutrition Diagnosis (one or more must be present)
Biochemical Data	• Hypoglycemia or hyperglycemia documented on regular basis when compared with goal of maintaining glucose levels at or below 140 mg/dL throughout the day
Anthropometric Measurements	
Physical Examination Findings	

INAPPROPRIATE INTAKE OF TYPES OF CARBOHYDRATES (SPECIFY) (NI-53.3)

Food/Nutrition History	Reports or observations of: • Diarrhea in response to high refined carbohydrate intake • Economic constraints that limit availability of appropriate foods • Carbohydrate intake that is different from recommended types • Allergic reactions to certain carbohydrate foods or food groups • Limited knowledge of carbohydrate composition of foods or of carbohydrate metabolism
Client History	• Conditions associated with a diagnosis or treatment, e.g., diabetes mellitus, obesity, metabolic syndrome, hypoglycemia • Chronic use of medications that cause altered glucose levels, e.g., steroids, antidepressants, antipsychotics

References:

1. Bowman BA, Russell RM. *Present Knowledge in Nutrition*. 8th ed. Washington, DC: ILSI Press, 2001.
2. Clement S, Braithwaite SS, Magee MF, Ahmann A, Smith EP, Schafer RG, Hirsch IB, American Diabetes Association Diabetes in Hospitals Writing Committee. Management of diabetes in hospitals. *Diabetes Care*. 2004;27:553-592.
3. Franz MJ, Bantle JP, Beebe CA, Brunzell JD, Chiasson J-L, Garg A, Holzmeister LA, Hoogwerf B, Mayer-Davis E, Mooradian AD, Purnell JQ, Wheeler M: Technical review. Evidence-based nutrition principles and recommendations for the treatment and prevention of diabetes and related complications. *Diabetes Care* 2002;202:148-198.
4. Sheard NF, Clark NG, Brand-Miller JC, Franz MJ, Pi-Sunyer FX, Mayer-Davis E, Kulkarni K, Geil P. A statement by the American Diabetes Association. Dietary carbohydrate (amount and type) in the prevention and management of diabetes. *Diabetes Car.e* 2004;27:2266-2271.
5. Gross LS, Li L, Ford ES, Liu S. Increased consumption of refined carbohydrates and epidemic or type 2 diabetes in the United States: an ecologic assessment. *Am J Clin Nutr* 2004;79:774-779.
6. French S, Lin B-H, Gutherie JF. National trends in soft drink consumption among children and adolescents age 6 to17 years: prevalence, amounts, and sources, 1977/1978 to 1994/1998. *J Am Diet Assoc* 2003.103L1326-1331,
7. National Academy of Sciences, Institute of Medicine. *Dietary Reference Intakes for Energy, Carbohydrate, Fiber, Fat, Fatty Acids, Cholesterol, Protein, and Amino Acids*. Washington, DC: National Academy Press; 2002.
8. Teff KL, Elliott SS, Tschöp M, Kieffer TJ, Rader D, Heiman M, Townsend RR, Keim NL, D'Alessio D, Havel PJ. Dietary fructose reduces circulating insulin and leptin, attenuates postprandial suppression of ghrelin, and increases triglycerides in women. *J Clin Endocrinol Meta.b* 2004;89:2963-2972.
9. The Expert Committee on the Diagnosis and Classification of Diabetes Mellitus. Diagnosis and classification of diabetes mellitus. *Diabetes Care*. 2004;27:pS5-pS10.

INCONSISTENT CARBOHYDRATE INTAKE (NI-53.4)

Definition

Inconsistent timing of carbohydrate intake throughout the day, day-to-day, or a pattern of carbohydrate intake that is not consistent with recommended pattern based upon physiologic or medication needs

Etiology *(Cause/Contributing Risk Factors)*

Factors gathered during the nutrition assessment process that contribute to the existence or the maintenance of pathophysiological, psychosocial, situational, developmental, cultural, and/or environmental problems:

- Physiologic causes requiring careful timing and consistency in the amount of carbohydrate, e.g., diabetes mellitus, hypoglycemia
- Cultural, religious practices, or lifestyle factors that interfere with the ability to regulate timing of carbohydrate consumption
- Food- and nutrition-related knowledge deficit, e.g., inability to access sufficient information concerning more appropriate timing of carbohydrate intake
- Food and nutrition compliance limitations, e.g., lack of willingness or failure to modify carbohydrate timing in response to recommendations from a dietitian, physician, or caregiver
- Psychological causes, e.g., depression or disordered eating

Signs/Symptoms *(Defining Characteristics)*

A typical cluster of subjective and objective signs and symptoms gathered during the nutrition assessment process that provide evidence that a problem exists; quantify the problem and describe its severity.

Nutrition Assessment Category	Potential Indicators of this Nutrition Diagnosis (one or more must be present)
Biochemical Data	• Hypoglycemia or hyperglycemia documented on regular basis associated with inconsistent carbohydrate intake • Wide variations in blood glucose levels
Anthropometric Measurements	
Physical Examination Findings	
Food/Nutrition History	Reports or observations of: • Economic constraints that limit availability of appropriate foods • Carbohydrate intake that is different from recommended types or ingested on an irregular basis

INCONSISTENT CARBOHYDRATE INTAKE (NI-53.4)

Client History	• Conditions associated with a diagnosis or treatment, e.g., diabetes mellitus, obesity, metabolic syndrome, hypoglycemia • Use of insulin or insulin secretagogues • Chronic use of medications that cause altered glucose levels, e.g., steroids, antidepressants, antipsychotics

References:

1. Bowman BA, Russell RM. *Present Knowledge in Nutrition.* 8th ed. Washington, DC: ILSI Press;2001.
2. Clement S, Braithwaite SS, Magee MF, Ahmann A, Smith EP, Schafer RG, Hirsch IB, American Diabetes Association Diabetes in Hospitals Writing Committee. Management of diabetes in hospitals. *Diabetes Care.* 2004;27:553-592.
3. Cryer PE, Davis SN, Shamoon H. Technical review. Hypoglycemia in diabetes. *Diabetes Care.* 2003;26:1902-1912.
4. Franz MJ, Bantle JP, Beebe CA, Brunzell JD, Chiasson J-L, Garg A, Holzmeister LA, Hoogwerf B, Mayer-Davis E, Mooradian AD, Purnell JQ, Wheeler M. Technical review. Evidence-based nutrition principles and recommendations for the treatment and prevention of diabetes and related complications. *Diabetes Care.* 2002;202:148-198.
5. National Academy of Sciences, Institute of Medicine. *Dietary Reference Intakes for Energy, Carbohydrate, Fiber, Fat, Fatty Acids, Cholesterol, Protein, and Amino Acids.* Washington, DC: National Academy Press; 2002.
6. Rabasa-Lhoret R, Garon J, Langelier H, Poisson D, Chiasson J-L: The effects of meal carbohydrate content on insulin requirements in type 1 patients with diabetes treated intensively with the basal bolus (ultralente-regular) insulin regimen. *Diabetes Care* 1999;22:667-673.
7. Savoca MR, Miller CK, Ludwig DA. Food habits are related to glycemic control among people with type 2 diabetes mellitus. *J Am Diet Assoc.* 2004;104:560-566.
8. The Expert Committee on the Diagnosis and Classification of Diabetes Mellitus. Diagnosis and classification of diabetes mellitus. *Diabetes Care.* 2004;27:S5-S10.
9. Wolever TMS, Hamad S, Chiasson J-L, Josse RG, Leiter LA, Rodger NW, Ross SA, Ryan EA. Day-to-day consistency in amount and source of carbohydrate intake associated with improved glucose control in type 1 diabetes. *J Am Coll Nutr.* 1999;18:242-247.

INADEQUATE FIBER INTAKE (NI-53.5)

Definition

Lower intake of fiber-containing foods or substances compared to established reference standards or recommendations based upon physiological needs

Etiology (*Cause/Contributing Risk Factors*)

Factors gathered during the nutrition assessment process that contribute to the existence or the maintenance of pathophysiological, psychosocial, situational, developmental, cultural, and/or environmental problems:

- Lack of access to fiber-containing foods
- Food- and nutrition-related knowledge deficit
- Psychological causes, e.g., depression or disordered eating
- Prolonged adherence to a low-fiber or low-residue diet
- Difficulty chewing or swallowing high-fiber foods
- Economic constraints that limit availability of appropriate foods
- Inability or unwillingness to purchase or consume fiber-containing foods
- Inappropriate food preparation practices, e.g., reliance on overprocessed, overcooked foods

Signs/Symptoms (*Defining Characteristics*)

A typical cluster of subjective and objective signs and symptoms gathered during the nutrition assessment process that provide evidence that a problem exists; quantify the problem and describe its severity.

Nutrition Assessment Category	Potential Indicators of this Nutrition Diagnosis (one or more must be present)
Biochemical Data	
Anthropometric Measurements	
Physical Examination Findings	
Food/Nutrition History	Reports or observations of: • Insufficient intake of fiber when compared to recommended amounts (38 g/day for men and 25 g/day for women; 21 g/d for women >50 years and 31 g/d for men >50 years)

INADEQUATE FIBER INTAKE (NI-53.5)

Client History	• Conditions associated with a diagnosis or treatment, e.g., ulcer disease, inflammatory bowel disease, or short bowel syndrome treated with a low-fiber diet • Low stool volume

References:

1. DiPalma JA. Current treatment options for chronic constipation. *Rev Gastroenterol Disord.* 2004;2:S34-S42.
2. Higgins PD, Johanson JF. Epidemiology of constipation in North America: a systematic review. *Am J Gastroenterol.* 2004;99:750-759.
3. Lembo A, Camilieri M. Chronic constipation. *New Engl J Med.* 2003;349:360-368.
4. National Academy of Sciences, Institute of Medicine. *Dietary Reference Intakes for Energy, Carbohydrate, Fiber, Fat, Fatty Acids, Cholesterol, Protein, and Amino Acids.* Washington, DC: National Academy Press; 2002.
5. Talley NJ. Definition, epidemiology, and impact of chronic constipation. *Rev Gastroenterol Disord.* 2004;2:S3-S10.

EXCESSIVE FIBER INTAKE (NI-53.6)

Definition

Higher intake of fiber-containing foods or substances compared to recommendations based upon patient/client condition

Etiology *(Cause/Contributing Risk Factors)*

Factors gathered during the nutrition assessment process that contribute to the existence or the maintenance of pathophysiological, psychosocial, situational, developmental, cultural, and/or environmental problems:

- Food- and nutrition-related knowledge deficit about desirable quantities of fiber for individual condition
- Harmful beliefs or attitudes about food or nutrition-related topics, e.g., obsession with bowel frequency and habits
- Lack of knowledge about appropriate fiber intake for condition
- Poor dentition, GI stricture or dysmotility
- Food preparation or eating patterns that involve only high-fiber foods to the exclusion of other nutrient-dense foods

Signs/Symptoms *(Defining Characteristics)*

A typical cluster of subjective and objective signs and symptoms gathered during the nutrition assessment process that provide evidence that a problem exists; quantify the problem and describe its severity.

Nutrition Assessment Category	Potential Indicators of this Nutrition Diagnosis (one or more must be present)
Biochemical Data	
Anthropometric Measurements	
Physical Examination Findings	
Food/Nutrition History	Reports or observations of: • Fiber intake higher than tolerated or generally recommended for current medical condition
Client History	• Conditions associated with a diagnosis or treatment, e.g., ulcer disease, irritable bowel syndrome, inflammatory bowel disease, short bowel syndrome, diverticulitis, obstructive constipation, prolapsing hemorrhoids, gastrointestinal stricture, eating disorders, or mental illness with obsessive-compulsive tendencies • Nausea, vomiting, excessive flatulence, diarrhea, abdominal cramping, high stool volume or frequency that causes discomfort to the individual, obstruction, phytobezoar

EXCESSIVE FIBER INTAKE (NI-53.6)

References:

1. DiPalma JA. Current treatment options for chronic constipation. *Rev Gastroenterol Disord.* 2004;2:S34-S42.
2. Higgins PD, Johanson JF. Epidemiology of constipation in North America: a systematic review. *Am J Gastroenterol.* 2004;99:750-759.
3. Lembo A, Camilieri M. Chronic constipation. *New Engl J Med.* 2003;349:360-368.
4. National Academy of Sciences, Institute of Medicine. *Dietary Reference Intakes for Energy, Carbohydrate, Fiber, Fat, Fatty Acids, Cholesterol, Protein, and Amino Acids.* Washington, DC: National Academy Press; 2002.
5. Position of the American Dietetic Association: Health implications of dietary fiber. *J Am Diet Assoc.* 2002;102:993-1000.
6. Talley NJ. Definition, epidemiology, and impact of chronic constipation. *Rev Gastroenterol Disord.* 2004;2:S3-S10.
7. van den Berg H, van der Gaag M, Hendriks H. Influence of lifestyle on vitamin bioavailability. *Int J Vitam Nutr Res.* 2002;72:53-55.
8. Wald A. Irritable bowel syndrome. *Curr Treat Options Gastroenterol.* 1999;2:13-19.

INADEQUATE VITAMIN INTAKE (SPECIFY) (NI-54.1)

Definition

Lower intake of vitamin-containing foods or substances compared to established reference standards or recommendations based upon physiological needs

Etiology *(Cause/Contributing Risk Factors)*

Factors gathered during the nutrition assessment process that contribute to the existence or the maintenance of pathophysiological, psychosocial, situational, developmental, cultural, and/or environmental problems:

- Physiologic causes, e.g., increased nutrient needs due to prolonged catabolic illness, disease state, malabsorption, or medications
- Lack of access to food, e.g., economic constraints, cultural or religious practices, restricting food given to elderly and/or children
- Food- and nutrition-related knowledge deficit concerning food sources of vitamins
- Psychological causes, e.g., depression or eating disorders

Signs/Symptoms *(Defining Characteristics)*

A typical cluster of subjective and objective signs and symptoms gathered during the nutrition assessment process that provide evidence that a problem exists; quantify the problem and describe its severity.

INADEQUATE VITAMIN INTAKE (SPECIFY) (NI-54.1)

Nutrition Assessment Category	Potential Indicators of this Nutrition Diagnosis (one or more must be present)*
Biochemical Data	• Vitamin A: serum retinol: < 10 µg/dL (0.35 µmol/L) • Vitamin C : plasma concentrations < 0.2 mg/dL (11.4 µmol/L) • Vitamin D: ionized calcium < 3.9 mg/dL (0.98 mmol/L) with elevated parathyroid hormone, normal serum calcium, and serum phosphorus < 2.6 mg/dL (0.84 mmol/L) • Vitamin E: plasma alpha-tocopherol < 18 µmol/g (41.8 µmol/L) • Vitamin K: elevated prothrombin time; altered INR (without anti-coagulation therapy) • Thiamin: erythrocyte transketolase activity > 1.20 µg/mL/h • Riboflavin – erythrocyte glutathione reductase > 1.2 IU/gm hemoglobin • Niacin: N'methyl-nicotinamide excretion < 5.8 µmol/day • Vitamin B6: plasma pryrdoxal 5'phosphate <5 ng/mL (20 nmol/L) • Vitamin B12: serum concentration < 24.4 ng/dL (180 pmol/L); elevated homocysteine • Folic acid: serum concentration < 0.3 µg/dL (7 nmol/L); red cell folate < 315 nmol/L
Anthropometric Measurements	
Physical Exam Findings	• Vitamin A: night blindness, Bitot's spots, xeropthalmia, follicular hyperkeratosis • Vitamin C: follicular hyperkeratosis, petichiae, ecchymosis, coiled hairs, inflamed and bleeding gums, perifolicular hemorrhages, joint effusions, arthralgia, and impaired wound healing • Vitamin D: widening at ends of long bones, rachitic rosary in children, rickets, osteomalacia • Riboflavin: sore throat, hyperemia, edema of pharyngeal and oral mucous membranes, cheilosis, angular stomatitis, glossitis, seborrheic dermatitis, and normochromic, normocytic anemia with pure erythrocyte cytoplasia of the bone marrow • Niacin: symmetrical, pigmented rash on areas exposed to sunlight, bright red tongue, pellagra • Vitamin B6: seborrheic dermatitis, stomatitis, cheilosis, glossitis, confusion, depression • Vitamin B12: tingling and numbness in extremities, diminished vibratory and position sense, motor disturbances including gait disturbances

* To convert conventional units to *le Systeme Internationale d'Unites (SI)*, Jays Clinical Services, Clinical Laboratory Software and Consulting web site used. Web site address: http://dwjay.tripod.com/conversion.html . Accessed August 12, 2005. See Young DS (Reference #5) for printed factor conversions.

INADEQUATE VITAMIN INTAKE (SPECIFY) (NI-54.1)

Food/Nutrition History	Reports or observations of: • Dietary history reflects inadequate intake of foods containing specific vitamins as compared to requirements or recommended level • Dietary history reflects excessive consumption of foods that do not contain available vitamins, e.g., overprocessed, overcooked, or improperly stored foods
Client History	• Prolonged use of substances known to increase vitamin requirements or reduce vitamin absorption • Conditions associated with a diagnosis or treatment, e.g., malabsorption as a result of celiac disease, short bowel syndrome, or inflammatory bowel • Certain environmental conditions, e.g., infants exclusively fed breast milk with limited exposure to sunlight (vitamin D)

References:

1. National Academy of Sciences, Institute of Medicine. *Dietary Reference Intakes for Vitamin A, Vitamin K, Arsenic, Boron, Chromium, Copper, Iodine, Iron, Manganese, Molybdenum, Nickel, Silicon, Vanadium, and Zinc*. Washington, DC: National Academy Press; 2000.
2. National Academy of Sciences, Institute of Medicine. *Dietary Reference Intakes for Thiamine, Riboflavin, Niacin, Vitamin B6, Folate, Vitamin B12, Pantothenic Acid, Biotin, and Choline* Washington, DC: National Academy Press; 2000.
3. National Academy of Sciences, Institute of Medicine. *Dietary Reference Intakes for Vitamin C, Vitamin E, Selenium, and Carotenoids*. Washington, DC: National Academy Press; 2000.
4. National Academy of Sciences, Institute of Medicine. *Dietary Reference Intakes for Calcium, Phosphorus, Magnesium, Vitamin D, and Fluoride*. Washington, DC: National Academy Press; 1997.
5. Young DS. Implementation of SI units for clinical laboratory data, style specifications and conversion tables. *Ann Intern Med*. 1987;106:114-29. Reprinted, *J Nutr*. 1990;120:20-35.

EXCESSIVE VITAMIN INTAKE (SPECIFY) (NI-54.2)

Definition

Higher intake of vitamin-containing foods or substances compared to established reference standards or recommendations based upon physiological needs

Etiology *(Cause/Contributing Risk Factors)*

Factors gathered during the nutrition assessment process that contribute to the existence or the maintenance of pathophysiological, psychosocial, situational, developmental, cultural, and/or environmental problems:

- Physiologic causes, e.g., decreased nutrient needs due to prolonged immobility or chronic renal disease
- Access to foods and supplements in excess of needs, e.g., cultural or religious practices, inappropriate food and supplements given to pregnant women, elderly or children
- Food- and nutrition-related knowledge deficit concerning food and supplemental sources of vitamins
- Psychological causes, e.g., depression or eating disorders
- Accidental overdose from oral and supplemental forms, enteral or parenteral sources

Signs/Symptoms *(Defining Characteristics)*

A typical cluster of subjective and objective signs and symptoms gathered during the nutrition assessment process that provide evidence that a problem exists; quantify the problem and describe its severity.

Nutrition Assessment Category	Potential Indicators of this Nutrition Diagnosis (one or more must be present)*
Biochemical Data	• Vitamin D: ionized calcium > 5.4 mg/dL (1.35 mmol/L) with elevated parathyroid hormone, normal serum calcium, and serum phosphorus > 2.6 mg/dL (0.84 mmol/L) • Vitamin K: slowed prothrombin time or altered INR • Niacin: N-methyl nicotinamide excretion > 5.8 µmol/day • Vitamin B6: plasma pyridoxal 5'phosphate > 5 ng/mL (20 nmol/L) • Vitamin A: serum retinol concentration > 60 µg/dL (2.09µmol/L)
Anthropometric Measurements	

* To convert conventional units to *le Systeme Internationale d'Unites (SI)*, Jays Clinical Services, Clinical Laboratory Software and Consulting web site used. Web site address: http://dwjay.tripod.com/conversion.html . Accessed August 12, 2005. See Young DS (Reference #8) for printed factor conversions.

EXCESSIVE VITAMIN INTAKE (SPECIFY) (NI-54.2)

Physical Exam Findings	• Vitamin A: changes in the skin and mucous membranes; dry lips (cheilitis), early-dryness of the nasal mucosa and eyes; later-dryness, erythema, scaling and peeling of the skin, hair loss, and nail fragility. Headache, nausea, and vomiting. Infants may have bulging fontanelle; children may develop bone alterations. • Vitamin D: elevated serum calcium (hypercalcemia) and phosphorus (hyperphosphatemia) levels; calcification of soft tissues (calcinosis), including the kidney, lungs, heart, and even the tympanic membrane of the ear, which can result in deafness. Headache and nausea. Infants given excessive amounts of vitamin D may have gastrointestinal upset, bone fragility, and retarded growth. • Vitamin K: hemolytic anemia in adults or sever jaundice in infants have been noted on rare occasions • Niacin: histamine release which causes flushing, aggravation of asthma or liver disease
Food/Nutrition History	Reports or observations of: • History or measured intake reflects excessive intake of foods and supplements containing vitamins as compared to estimated requirements, including fortified cereals, meal replacements, vitamin-mineral supplements, other dietary supplements (e.g., fish liver oils or capsules), tube feeding, and/or parenteral solutions • Intake > Tolerable Upper Limits (UL) for vitamin A (as retinol ester, not as β-carotene) is 600 μg/d for infants and toddlers; 900 μg/d for children 4-8 yrs, 1,700 μg/d for children 9-13 yrs, 2,800 μg/d for children 14-18 yrs, and 3,000 μg/d for adults • Intake greater than UL for vitamin D is 25 μg/day for infants and 50 μg/day for children and adults • Niacin: clinical, high-dose niacinamide (NA) use of 1 to 2 g, three times per day can have side effects
Client History	• Conditions associated with a diagnosis or treatment, e.g., chronic liver or kidney diseases, heart failure, cancer

References:

1. Allen LH, Haskell M. Estimating the potential for vitamin A toxicity in women and young children. *J Nutr.* 2002;132:S2907-S2919.
2. Croquet V, Pilette C, Lespine A, Vuillemin E, Rousselet MC, Oberti F, Saint Andre JP, Periquet B, Francois S, Ifrah N, Cales P. Hepatic hyper-vitaminosis A: importance of retinyl ester level determination. *Eur J Gastroenterol Hepatol.* 2000;12:361-364.
3. Krasinski SD, Russell RM, Otradovec CL, Sadowski JA, Hartz SC, Jacob RA, McGandy RB. Relationship of vitamin A and vitamin E intake to fasting plasma retinol, retinol-binding protein, retinyl esters, carotene, alpha-tocopherol, and cholesterol among elderly people and young adults: increased plasma retinyl esters among vitamin A-supplement users. *Am J Clin Nutr.* 1989;49:112-120.
4. National Academy of Sciences, Institute of Medicine. *Dietary Reference Intakes for Vitamin A, Vitamin K, Arsenic, Boron, Chromium, Copper, Iodine, Iron, Manganese, Molybdenum, Nickel, Silicon, Vanadium, and Zinc.* Washington, DC: National Academy Press; 2000.
5. National Academy of Sciences, Institute of Medicine. *Dietary Reference Intakes for Thiamine, Riboflavin, Niacin, Vitamin B6, Folate, Vitamin B12, Pantothenic Acid, Biotin, and Choline* Washington, DC: National Academy Press; 2000.
6. National Academy of Sciences, Institute of Medicine. *Dietary Reference Intakes for Vitamin C, Vitamin E, Selenium, and Carotenoids.* Washington, DC: National Academy Press;2000.
7. Russell RM. New views on RDAs for older adults. *J Am Diet Assoc.* 1997;97:515-518.
8. Young DS. Implementation of SI units for clinical laboratory data, style specifications and conversion tables. *Ann Intern Med.* 1987;106:114-29. Reprinted, *J Nutr.* 1990;120:20-35..

INADEQUATE MINERAL INTAKE (SPECIFY) (NI-55.1)

Definition

Lower intake of mineral-containing foods or substances compared to established reference standards or recommendations based upon physiological needs

Etiology (*Cause/Contributing Risk Factors*)

Factors gathered during the nutrition assessment process that contribute to the existence or the maintenance of pathophysiological, psychosocial, situational, developmental, cultural, and/or environmental problems:

- Physiologic causes, e.g., increased nutrient needs due to prolonged catabolic illness, malabsorption, hyperexcretion, nutrient/drug and nutrient/nutrient interaction, growth and maturation
- Lack of access to food, e.g., economic constraints, cultural or religious practices, restricting food given to elderly and/or children
- Food- and nutrition-related knowledge deficit concerning food sources of minerals; misdiagnosis of lactose intolerance/lactase deficiency; perception of conflicting nutrition messages from health professionals, inappropriate reliance on supplements
- Psychological causes, e.g., depression or eating disorders
- Environmental causes, e.g., inadequately tested nutrient bioavailability of fortified foods, beverages and supplements, inappropriate marketing of fortified foods/beverages/supplements as a substitute for natural food source of nutrient(s)

Signs/Symptoms (*Defining Characteristics*)

A typical cluster of subjective and objective signs and symptoms gathered during the nutrition assessment process that provide evidence that a problem exists; quantify the problem and describe its severity.

Nutrition Assessment Category	Potential Indicators of this Nutrition Diagnosis (one or more must be present)*
Biochemical Data	• Calcium: bone mineral content (BMC) below the young adult mean. Hypocalciuria, serum 25(OH)D < 32 ng/mL • Phosphorus < 2.6 mg/dL (0.84 mmol/L) • Magnesium < 1.8 mg/dL (0.7 mmol/L) • Iron: hemoglobin < 130 g/L (males); < 120 g /L (females) • Iodine: urinary excretion < 100 µg /L (788 nmol/L) • Copper : serum copper < 64 µg /dL (10 µmol/L)
Anthropometric Measurements	• Height loss

* To convert conventional units to *le Systeme Internationale d'Unites (SI)*, Jays Clinical Services, Clinical Laboratory Software and Consulting web site used. Web site address: http://dwjay.tripod.com/conversion.html . Accessed August 12, 2005. See Young DS (Reference #5) for printed factor conversions.

INADEQUATE MINERAL INTAKE (SPECIFY) (NI-55.1)

Physical Exam Findings	• Calcium: diminished bone mineral density, hypertension, polycystic ovary syndrome, premenstrual syndrome, kidney stones, colon polyps, obesity
Food/Nutrition History	Observations/reports of insufficient mineral intake from diet compared to recommended intake: • Food avoidance and/or elimination of whole food group(s) from diet • Lack of interest in food • Inappropriate food choices and/or chronic dieting behavior • Excessive Na intake, inadequate vitamin D intake/exposure
Client History	• Conditions associated with a diagnosis or treatment of, e.g., malabsorption as a result of celiac disease, short bowel syndrome, or inflammatory bowel disease • Other significant medical diagnoses and therapies • Estrogen status • Geographic latitude and history of UVB exposure/use of sunscreen • Change in living environment/independence • Use of popular press/internet as source of medical and/or nutrition information

References:

1. Appel LJ, Moore TJ, Obarzanek E, Vollmer WM, Svetkey LP, Sacks FM, Bray GA, Vogt TM, Cutler JA, Windhauser MM, Lin P-H, Karanja N. A clinical trial of the effects of dietary patterns on blood pressure. *N Engl J Med.* 1997;336:1117-1124.
2. Heaney RP. Role of dietary sodium in osteoporosis. *Am J Clin Nutr* (in press) 2005.
3. Heaney RP. Nutrients, interactions, and foods. The importance of source. In: Burckhardt P, Dawson-Hughes B, Heaney RP, eds. *Nutritional Aspects of Osteoporosis.* 2nd ed. San Diego, Calif: Elsevier. 2004:61-76.
4. Heaney, RP. Nutrients, interactions, and foods. Serum 25-hydroxy-vitamin D and the health of the calcium economy. In Burckhardt P, Dawson-Hughes B, Heaney RP, eds. *Nutritional Aspects of Osteoporosis.* 2nd ed. San Diego, Calif: Elsevier. 2004:227-244.
5. Heaney RP, Rafferty K, Bierman J. Not all calcium-fortified beverages are equal. *Nutr Today.* 2005;40:39-41.
6. Heaney RP, Dowell MS, Hale CA, Bendich A. Calcium absorption varies within the reference range for serum 25-hydroxyvitamin D. *J Am Coll Nutr.* 2003;22:142-146.
7. Heaney RP, Dowell MS, Rafferty K, Bierman J. Bioavailability of the calcium in fortified soy imitation milk, with some observations on method. *Am J Clin Nutr.* 2000;71:1166-1169.
8. Holick MF. Functions of vitamin D: importance for prevention of common cancers, type I diabetes and heart disease. In: Burckhardt P, Dawson-Hughes B, Heaney RP, eds. *Nutritional Aspects of Osteoporosis.* 2nd ed. San Diego, Calif: Elsevier;2004:181-201.
9. Massey LK, Whiting SJ. Dietary salt, urinary calcium, and bone loss. *J Bone Miner Res.* 1996 ;11:731-736.
10. Suaraz FL, Savaiano D, Arbisi P, Levitt MD. Tolerance to the daily ingestion of two cups of milk by individuals claiming lactose intolerance. *Am J Clin Nutr.* 1997;65:1502-1506.
11. Thys- Jacobs S, Donovan D, Papadopoulos A, Sarrel P. Bilezikian JP. Vitamin D and calcium dysregulation in the polycystic ovarian syndrome. *Steroids.* 1999;64:430-435.
12. Thys-Jacobs S, Starkey P, Bernstein D, Tian J. Calcium carbonate and the premenstrual syndrome: Effects on premenstrual and menstrual symptomatology. *Am J Obstet Gynecol.* 1998;179:444-452.
13. Young DS. Implementation of SI units for clinical laboratory data, style specifications and conversion tables. *Ann Intern Med.* 1987;106:114-29. Reprinted, *J Nutr.* 1990;120:20-35.
14. Zemel MB, Thompson W, Milstead A, Morris K, Campbell P. Calcium and dairy acceleration of weight and fat loss during energy restriction in obese adults. *Obesity Res.* 2004;12:582-590.

EXCESSIVE MINERAL INTAKE (SPECIFY) (NI-55.2)

Definition

Higher intake of mineral from foods, supplements, medications or water, compared to established reference standards or recommendations based upon physiological needs

Etiology (*Cause/Contributing Risk Factors*)

Factors gathered during the nutrition assessment process that contribute to the existence or the maintenance of pathophysiological, psychosocial, situational, developmental, cultural, and/or environmental problems:

- Food- and nutrition-related knowledge deficit
- Harmful beliefs/attitudes about food, nutrition, and nutrition-related topics
- Food faddism
- Accidental over-supplementation
- Overconsumption of a limited variety of foods
- Lack of knowledge about management of diagnosed genetic disorder that alters mineral homeostasis such as hemochromotosis (iron), Wilson's Disease (copper)
- Lack of knowledge about management of diagnosed disease state that requires mineral restriction such as cholestatic liver disease (copper and manganese) and renal insufficiency (phosphorus, magnesium, potassium)

Signs/Symptoms (*Defining Characteristics*)

A typical cluster of subjective and objective signs and symptoms gathered during the nutrition assessment process that provide evidence that a problem exists; quantify the problem and describe its severity.

EXCESSIVE MINERAL INTAKE (SPECIFY) (NI-55.2)

Nutrition Assessment Category	Potential Indicators of this Nutrition Diagnosis (one or more must be present)
Biochemical Data	Changes in appropriate laboratory values, such as: • ↑ TSH (iodine supplementation) • ↓ HDL (zinc supplementation) • ↑ serum ferritin and transferrin saturation (iron overload) • Hyperphosphatemia • Hypermagnesemia
Anthropometric Measurements	
Physical Exam Findings	• Hair and nail changes (selenium)
Food/Nutrition History	Reports or observations of: • High intake of foods or supplements containing minerals compared to DRIs • Decreased appetite (zinc supplementation)
Client History	• GI disturbances (iron, magnesium, copper, zinc, selenium) • Copper-deficiency anemia (zinc) • Liver damage (copper, iron), enamel or skeletal fluorosis (fluoride)

References:

1. Bowman BA, Russell RM, eds. *Present Knowledge in Nutrition.* 8th ed. Washington, DC: ILSI Press; 2001.
2. National Academy of Sciences, Institute of Medicine. *Dietary Reference Intakes for Vitamin A, Vitamin K, Arsenic, Boron, Chromium, Copper, Iodine, Iron, Manganese, Molybdenum, Nickel, Silicon, Vanadium, Zinc.* Washington, DC: National Academy Press; 2001.
3. National Academy of Sciences, Institute of Medicine. *Dietary Reference Intakes for Calcium, Phosphorus, Magnesium, Vitamin D, and Fluoride.* Washington, DC: National Academy Press; 1997.
4. Position of the American Dietetic Association: Food and nutrition misinformation. *J Am Diet Assoc.* 2002;102:260-266.

SWALLOWING DIFFICULTY (NC-1.1)

Definition

Impaired movement of food and liquid from the mouth to the stomach

Etiology (*Cause/Contributing Risk Factors*)

Factors gathered during the nutrition assessment process that contribute to the existence or the maintenance of pathophysiological, psychosocial, situational, developmental, cultural, and/or environmental problems:

- Mechanical causes, e.g., inflammation, surgery, stricture, or oral, pharyngeal and esophageal tumors
- Motor causes, e.g., neurological or muscular disorders, such as, cerebral palsy, stroke, multiple sclerosis, scleroderma, prematurity

Signs/Symptoms (*Defining Characteristics*)

A typical cluster of subjective and objective signs and symptoms gathered during the nutrition assessment process that provide evidence that a problem exists; quantify the problem and describe its severity.

Nutrition Assessment Category	Potential Indicators of this Nutrition Diagnosis (one or more must be present)
Biochemical Data	
Anthropometric Measurements	
Physical Exam Findings	• Evidence of dehydration, e.g., dry mucous membranes, poor skin turgor
Food/Nutrition History	Observations or reports of: • Coughing, choking, prolonged chewing, pouching of food, regurgitation, facial expression changes during eating, prolonged feeding time, drooling, noisy wet upper airway sounds, feeling of "food getting stuck," pain while swallowing • Decreased food intake • Avoidance of foods • Mealtime resistance
Client History	• Conditions associated with a diagnosis or treatment of dysphagia, achalasia • Radiological findings, e.g., abnormal swallowing studies • Repeated upper respiratory infections and or pneumonia

Reference:

1. Braunwald E, Fauci AS, Kasper DL, Hauser SL, Longo DL, Jameson JL, eds. *Harrison's Principles of Internal Medicine.* 15th ed. New York, NY: McGraw-Hill,.2001.

CHEWING (MASTICATORY) DIFFICULTY (NC-1.2)

Definition

Impaired ability to bite or chew food in preparation for swallowing

Etiology *(Cause/Contributing Risk Factors)*

Factors gathered during the nutrition assessment process that contribute to the existence or the maintenance of pathophysiological, psychosocial, situational, developmental, cultural, and/or environmental problems:

- Craniofacial malformations
- Oral surgery
- Neuromuscular dysfunction
- Partial or complete edentulism
- Soft tissue disease (primary or oral manifestations of a systemic disease)
- Xerostomia

Signs/Symptoms *(Defining Characteristics)*

A typical cluster of subjective and objective signs and symptoms gathered during the nutrition assessment process that provide evidence that a problem exists; quantify the problem and describe its severity.

Nutrition Assessment Category	Potential Indicators of this Nutrition Diagnosis (one or more must be present)
Biochemical Data	
Anthropometric Measurements	
Physical Exam Findings	• Missing teeth • Alterations in cranial nerves V, VII, IX, X, XII • Dry or cracked lips, tongue • Oral lesions • Impaired tongue movement • Ill-fitting dentures or broken dentures

CHEWING (MASTICATORY) DIFFICULTY (NC-1.2)

Food/Nutrition History	Reports or observations of: • Decreased intake of food • Alterations in food intake from usual • Decreased intake or avoidance of food difficult to form into a bolus, e.g., nuts, whole pieces of meat, poultry, fish, fruits, vegetables • Avoidance of foods of age-appropriate texture • Spitting food out or prolonged feeding time
Client History	• Conditions associated with a diagnosis or treatment, e.g., alcoholism; Alzheimer's; head, neck or pharyngeal cancer;, cerebral palsy; cleft lip/palate; oral soft tissue infections (e.g., candidiasis, leukoplakia); lack of developmental readiness; oral manifestations of systemic disease (e.g., rheumatoid arthritis, lupus, Crohn's disease, penphigus vulgaris, HIV, diabetes) • Recent major oral surgery • Wired jaw • Chemotherapy with oral side effects • Radiation therapy to oral cavity

References:

1. Bailey R, Ledikwe JH, Smiciklas-Wright H, Mitchell DC, Jensen GL. Persistent oral health problems associated with comorbidity and impaired diet quality in older adults. *J Am Diet Assoc.* 2004;104:1273-1276.
2. Martin WE. Oral health in the elderly. In: Chernoff R, ed.. *Geriatric Nutrition.* 2nd ed. Gaithersburg, Maryl: Aspen Publishers; 1999:107-169.
3. Dormenval V, Mojon P, Budtz-Jorgensen E. Association between self-assessed masticatory ability, nutritional status and salivary flow rate in hospitalized elderly. *Oral Dis.* 1999;5:32-38.
4. Hildebrand GH, Dominguez BL, Schork MA, Loesche WJ. Functional units, chewing, swallowing and food avoidance among the elderly. *J Prosthet Dent.* 1997;77:585-595.
5. Hirano H, Ishiyama N, Watanabe I, Nasu I. Masticatory ability in relation to oral status and general health in aging. *J Nutr Health Aging.* 1999;3:48-52.
6. Huhmann M, Touger-Decker R, Byham-Gray L, O'Sullivan-Maillet J, Von Hagen S. Comparison of dysphagia screening by a registered dietitian in acute stroke patients to speech language pathologist's evaluation. *Top Clin Nutr.* 2004;19:239-249.
7. Kademani D, Glick M. Oral ulcerations in individuals infected with human immunodeficiency virus: clinical presentations, diagnosis, management and relevance to disease progression. *Quintessence Int.*. 1998;29:1103-1108.
8. Keller HH, Ostbye T, Bright-See E. Predictors of dietary intake in Ontario seniors. *Can J Public Health.* 1997;88:303-309.
9. Krall E, Hayes C, Garcia R. How dentition status and masticatory function affect nutrient intake. *J Am Dent Assoc.* 1998;129:1261-1269.
10. Joshipura K, Willett WC, Douglass CW. The impact of edentulousness on food and nutrient intake. *J Am Dent Assoc.* 1996;127:459-467.
11. Mackle T, Touger-Decker R, O'Sullivan Maillet J, Holland B. Registered Dietitians' use of physical assessment parameters in practice. *J Am Diet Assoc.* 2004;103:1632-1638.
12. Mobley C, Saunders M. Oral health screening guidelines for nondental healthcare providers. *J Am Diet Assoc.* 1997;97:S123-126.
13. Morse, D. Oral and pharyngeal cancer. In: Touger-Decker R, Sirois D, Mobley C., eds. *Nutrition and Oral Medicine.* Totowa NJ: Humana Press. 2005.
14. Moynihan P, Butler T, Thomason J, Jepson N. Nutrient intake in partially dentate patients: the effect of prosthetic rehabilitation. *J Dent.* 2000;28:557-563.
15. Position of the American Dietetic Association: Oral health and nutrition. *J Am Diet Assoc.* 2003;103:615-625.
16. Sayhoun NR, Lin CL, Krall E. Nutritional status of the older adult is associated with dentition status. *J Am Diet Assoc.* 2003;103:61-66.
18. Sheiham A, Steele JG. The impact of oral health on stated ability to eat certain foods; finding from the national diet and nutrition survey of older people in Great Britain. *Gerodontology.* 1999;16:11-20.
19. Ship J, Duffy V, Jones J, Langmore S. Geriatric oral health and its impact on eating. *J Am Geriatr Soc.* 1996;44:456-464.

CHEWING (MASTICATORY) DIFFICULTY (NC-1.2)

20. Touger-Decker R. Clinical and laboratory assessment of nutrition status. *Dent Clin North Am.*. 2003;47:259-278.
21. Touger-Decker R, Sirois D, Mobley C, eds. *Nutrition and Oral Medicine*. Totowa NJ: Humana Press. 2005
22. Walls AW, Steele JG, Sheiham A, Marcenes W, Moynihan PJ. Oral health and nutrition in older people. *J Public Health Dent.* 2000;60:304-307.

BREASTFEEDING DIFFICULTY (NC-1.3)

Definition

Inability to sustain infant nutrition through breastfeeding

Etiology (*Cause/Contributing Risk Factors*)

Factors gathered during the nutrition assessment process that contribute to the existence or the maintenance of pathophysiological, psychosocial, situational, developmental, cultural, and/or environmental problems:

Infant:
- Difficulty latching on, e.g., tight frenulum
- Poor sucking ability
- Oral pain
- Malnutrition/malabsorption
- Lethargy, sleepiness
- Irritability
- Swallowing difficulty

Mother:
- Painful breasts, nipples
- Breast or nipple abnormality
- Mastitis
- Perception of inadequate milk supply
- Lack of social, cultural, or environmental support

Signs/Symptoms (*Defining Characteristics*)

A typical cluster of subjective and objective signs and symptoms gathered during the nutrition assessment process that provide evidence that a problem exists; quantify the problem and describe its severity.

Nutrition Assessment Category	Potential Indicators of this Nutrition Diagnosis (one or more must be present)
Biochemical Data	• Laboratory evidence of dehydration in infant
Anthropometric Measurements	• Any weight loss or poor weight gain in infant
Physical Exam Findings	• Frenulum abnormality (infant)

BREASTFEEDING DIFFICULTY (NC-1.3)

Food/Nutrition History	Observations or reports of (infant): • Coughing • Crying, latching on and off, pounding on breasts • Decreased feeding frequency/duration, early cessation of feeding, and/or feeding resistance • Infant lethargy • Hunger, lack of satiety after feeding • Fewer than six wet diapers in 24 hours • Infant vomiting or diarrhea Observations or reports of (mother): • Small amount of milk when pumping • Lack of confidence in ability to breastfeed • Doesn't hear infant swallowing • Concerns regarding mother's choice to breastfeed/lack of support • Insufficient knowledge of breastfeeding or infant hunger/satiety signals • Lack of facilities or accommodations at place of employment or in community for breastfeeding
Client History	• Conditions associated with a diagnosis or treatment (infant), e.g., cleft lip/palate, thrush, premature birth, malabsorption, infection • Conditions associated with a diagnosis or treatment (mother), e.g., mastitis, candidiasis, engorgement, history of breast surgery

References:

1. Barron SP, Lane HW, Hannan TE, Struempler B, Williams JC. Factors influencing duration of breast feeding among low-income women. *J Am Diet Assoc.* 1988;88:1557-1561.
2. Bryant C, Coreil J, D'Angelo SL, Bailey DFC, Lazarov MA. A strategy for promoting breastfeeding among economically disadvantaged women and adolescents. *NAACOG's Clin Issu Perinat Womens Health Nurs.* 1992;3:723-730.
3. Bentley ME, Caulfield LE, Gross SM, Bronner Y, Jensen J, Kessler LA, Paige DM. Sources of influence on intention to breastfeed among African-American women at entry to WIC. *J Hum Lact.* 1999;15:27-34.
4. Moreland JC, Lloyd L, Braun SB, Heins JN. A new teaching model to prolong breastfeeding among Latinos. *J Hum Lact.* 2000;16:337-341.
5. Position of the American Dietetic Association: Breaking the barriers to breastfeeding. *J Am Diet Assoc.* 2001;101:1213-1220.
6. Wooldrige MS, Fischer C. Colic, "overfeeding" and symptoms of lactose malabsorption in the breast-fed baby. *Lancet.* 1988;2:382-384.

ALTERED GASTROINTESTINAL (GI) FUNCTION (NC-1.4)

Definition

Changes in ability to digest or absorb nutrients

Etiology (*Cause/Contributing Risk Factors*)

Factors gathered during the nutrition assessment process that contribute to the existence or the maintenance of pathophysiological, psychosocial, situational, developmental, cultural, and/or environmental problems:

- Alterations in GI anatomical structure, e.g., gastric bypass, Roux en Y
- Changes in the GI tract motility, e.g., gastroparesis
- Compromised GI tract function, e.g., celiac disease, Crohn's disease, infection, radiation therapy
- Compromised function of related GI organs, e.g., pancreas, liver
- Decreased functional length of the GI tract, e.g., short bowel syndrome

Signs/Symptoms (*Defining Characteristics*)

A typical cluster of subjective and objective signs and symptoms gathered during the nutrition assessment process that provide evidence that a problem exists; quantify the problem and describe its severity.

Nutrition Assessment Category	Potential Indicators of this Nutrition Diagnosis (one or more must be present)
Biochemical Data	• Abnormal digestive enzyme and fecal fat studies • Abnormal hydrogen breath test, d-xylose test, stool culture, and gastric emptying and/or small bowel transit time
Anthropometric Measurements	• Wasting due to malnutrition in severe cases
Physical Exam Findings	• Decreased muscle mass • Abdominal distension • Increased (or sometimes decreased) bowel sounds

ALTERED GASTROINTESTINAL (GI) FUNCTION (NC-1.4)

Food/Nutrition History	Observations or reports of: • Avoidance or limitation of total intake or intake of specific foods/food groups due to GI symptoms, e.g., bloating, cramping, pain, diarrhea, steatorrhea (greasy, floating, foul-smelling stools) especially following ingestion of food • Food and nutrition-related knowledge deficit, e.g., lack of information, incorrect information or noncompliance with modified diet or medication schedule
Client History	• Anorexia, nausea, vomiting, diarrhea, steatorrhea, constipation, abdominal pain • Endoscopic or colonoscopic examination results, biopsy results • Conditions associated with a diagnosis or treatment, e.g., malabsorption, maldigestion, steatorrhea, constipation, diverticulitis, Crohn's disease, inflammatory bowel disease, cystic fibrosis, celiac disease, irritable bowel syndrome, infection • Surgical procedures, e.g., esophagectomy, dilatation, gastrectomy, vagotomy, gastric bypass, bowel resections

Reference:

1. Braunwald E, Fauci AS, Kasper DL, Hauser SL, Longo DL, Jameson JL, eds. *Harrison's Principles of Internal Medicine.* 15th ed. New York, NY: McGraw-Hill;2001.

IMPAIRED NUTRIENT UTILIZATION (NC-2.1)

Definition

Changes in ability to absorb or metabolize nutrients and bioactive substances

Etiology (*Cause/Contributing Risk Factors*)

Factors gathered during the nutrition assessment process that contribute to the existence or the maintenance of pathophysiological, psychosocial, situational, developmental, cultural, and/or environmental problems:

- Alterations in gastrointestinal anatomical structure
- Compromised function of the GI tract
- Compromised function of related GI organs, e.g., pancreas, liver
- Decreased functional length of the GI tract
- Metabolic disorders

Signs/Symptoms (*Defining Characteristics*)

A typical cluster of subjective and objective signs and symptoms gathered during the nutrition assessment process that provide evidence that a problem exists; quantify the problem and describe its severity.

Nutrition Assessment Category	Potential Indicators of this Nutrition Diagnosis (one or more must be present)
Biochemical Data	• Abnormal digestive enzyme and fecal fat studies • Abnormal hydrogen breath test, d-xylose test • Abnormal tests for inborn errors of metabolism
Anthropometric Measurements	• Weight loss of 5% in 1 month, 10% in 6 months • Growth stunting or failure
Physical Exam Findings	• Abdominal distension • Increased or decreased bowel sounds • Evidence of vitamin or mineral deficiency, e.g., glossitis, cheilosis, mouth lesions

IMPAIRED NUTRIENT UTILIZATION (NC-2.1)

Food/Nutrition History	Observations or reports of: • Avoidance or limitation of total intake or intake of specific foods/food groups due to GI symptoms, e.g., bloating, cramping, pain, diarrhea, steatorrhea (greasy, floating, foul-smelling stools) especially following ingestion of food
Client History	• Diarrhea, steatorrhea, abdominal pain • Endoscopic or colonoscopic examination results, biopsy results • Conditions associated with a diagnosis or treatment, e.g., malabsorption, maldigestion, cystic fibrosis, celiac disease, Crohn's disease, infection, radiation therapy, inborn errors of metabolism • Surgical procedures, e.g., gastric bypass, bowel resection

References:

1. Beyer P. Gastrointestinal disorders: Roles of nutrition and the dietetics practitioner. *J Am Diet Assoc.* 1998;98:272-277.
2. Position of the American Dietetic Association: Health implications of dietary fiber. *J Am Diet Assoc.* 2002;102:993-1000.

ALTERED NUTRITION-RELATED LABORATORY VALUES (SPECIFY) (NC-2.2)

Definition

Changes due to body composition, medications, body system or genetics, or changes in ability to eliminate byproducts of digestive and metabolic processes

Etiology (*Cause/Contributing Risk Factors*)

Factors gathered during the nutrition assessment process that contribute to the existence or the maintenance of pathophysiological, psychosocial, situational, developmental, cultural, and/or environmental problems:

- Kidney, liver, cardiac, endocrine, neurologic, and/or pulmonary dysfunction
- Other organ dysfunction that leads to biochemical changes:

Signs/Symptoms (*Defining Characteristics*)

A typical cluster of subjective and objective signs and symptoms gathered during the nutrition assessment process that provide evidence that a problem exists; quantify the problem and describe its severity.

Nutrition Assessment Category	Potential Indicators of this Nutrition Diagnosis (one or more must be present)
Biochemical Data	Findings such as: • Increased AST, ALT, T. bili, serum ammonia (liver disorders) • Abnormal BUN, Cr, K, phosphorus, glomerular filtration rate (GFR) (kidney disorders) • Altered pO_2 and pCO_2 (pulmonary disorders) • Abnormal serum lipids • Abnormal plasma glucose levels • Other findings of acute or chronic disorders that are abnormal and of nutritional origin or consequence
Anthropometric Measurements	• Rapid weight changes • Other anthropometric measures that are altered
Physical Exam Findings	• Jaundice, edema, ascites, itching (liver disorders) • Edema, shortness of breath (cardiac disorders) • Blue nail beds, clubbing (pulmonary disorders)

ALTERED NUTRITION-RELATED LABORATORY VALUES (SPECIFY) (NC-2.2)

Food/Nutrition History	Observations or reports of: • Anorexia, nausea, vomiting • Inability to consume full meals due to shortness of breath or abdominal distention • Intake of foods high in or overall excess intake of protein, potassium, phosphorus, sodium, fluid • Inadequate intake of micronutrients • Food- and nutrition-related knowledge deficit, e.g., lack of information, incorrect information or noncompliance with modified diet
Client History	• Conditions associated with a diagnosis or treatment of, e.g., renal or liver disease, alcoholism, cardio-pulmonary disorders

References:

1. Beto JA, Bansal VK. Medical nutrition therapy in chronic kidney failure: integrating clinical practice guidelines. *J Am Diet Assoc.* 2004;104:404-409.
2. Davern II TJ, Scharschmidt BF. Biochemical liver tests. In Feldman M, Scharschmidt BF, Sleisenger MH, eds. *Sleisenger and Fordtran's Gasrointestinal and Liver Disease, ed 6, vol 2.* Philadelphia, Pa: WB Saunders, 1998:1112-1122.
3. Durose CL, Holdsworth M, Watson V, Przygrodzka F. Knowledge of dietary restrictions and the medical consequences of noncompliance by patients on hemodialysis are not predictive of dietary compliance. *J Am Diet Assoc.* 2004;104:35-41.
4. Kasiske BL, Lakatua JD, Ma JZ, Louis TA. A meta-analysis of the effects of dietary protein restriction on the rate of decline in renal function. *Am J Kidney Dis.* 1998;31;954-961.
5. Knight EL, Stampfer MJ, Hankinson SE, Spiegelman D, Curhan GC. The impact of protein intake on renal function decline in women with normal renal function or mild renal insufficiency. *Ann Intern Med.* 2003;138:460-467.
6. Nakao T, Matsumoto, Okada T, Kanazawa Y, Yoshino M, Nagaoka Y, Takeguchi F. Nutritional management of dialysis patients: balancing among nutrient intake, dialysis dose, and nutritional status. *Am J Kidney Dis.* 2003;41:S133-S136.
7. National Kidney Foundation. Part 5. Evaluation of laboratory measurements for clinical assessment of kidney disease. *Am J Kidney Dis.* 2002;39:S76-S92.
8. National Kidney Foundation. Guideline 9. Association of level of GFR with nutritional status. *Am J Kidney Dis.* 2002;39:S128-S142.

FOOD-MEDICATION INTERACTION (NC-2.3)

Definition

Undesirable/harmful interaction(s) between food and over-the-counter (OTC) medications, prescribed medications, herbals, botanicals, and/or dietary supplements that diminishes, enhances, or alters effect of nutrients and/or medications

Etiology *(Cause/Contributing Risk Factors)*

Factors gathered during the nutrition assessment process that contribute to the existence or the maintenance of pathophysiological, psychosocial, situational, developmental, cultural, and/or environmental problems:

- Combined ingestion or administration of medication and food that results in undesirable/harmful interaction(s)

Signs/Symptoms *(Defining Characteristics)*

A typical cluster of subjective and objective signs and symptoms gathered during the nutrition assessment process that provide evidence that a problem exists; quantify the problem and describe its severity.

Nutrition Assessment Category	Potential Indicators of this Nutrition Diagnosis (one or more must be present)
Biochemical Data	• Alterations of biochemical tests based upon medication effect and patient/client condition
Anthropometric Measurements	• Alterations of anthropometric measurements based upon medication effect and patient/client conditions, e.g., weight gain and corticosteroids
Physical Exam Findings	

Food/Nutrition History	Observations or reports of:
	• Intake that is problematic or inconsistent with OTC, prescribed drugs, herbals, botanicals, or dietary supplements such as:
	  • fish oils and prolonged bleeding
	  • coumadin, vitamin K-rich foods
	  • high-fat diet while on cholesterol-lowering medications
	  • iron supplements, constipation and low-fiber diet
	• Intake that does not support replacement or mitigation of OTC, prescribed drugs, herbals, botanicals, or dietary supplements affects such as potassium-wasting diuretics
	• Changes in appetite or taste

FOOD-MEDICATION INTERACTION (NC-2.3)

Client History	• Multiple drugs (OTC, prescribed drugs, herbals, botanicals, or dietary supplements) that are known to have food medication interactions • Medications that require nutrient supplementation that can not be accomplished via food intake such as isoniazid and Vitamin B6

Reference:

1. Position of the American Dietetic Association: Integration of nutrition and pharmacotherapy. *J Am Diet Assoc.* 2003;103:1363-1370.

UNDERWEIGHT (NC-3.1)

Definition

Low body weight compared to established reference standards or recommendations

Etiology *(Cause/Contributing Risk Factors)*

Factors gathered during the nutrition assessment process that contribute to the existence or the maintenance of pathophysiological, psychosocial, situational, developmental, cultural, and/or environmental problems:

- Disordered eating pattern
- Excessive physical activity
- Harmful beliefs/attitudes about food, nutrition, and nutrition-related topics
- Inadequate energy intake
- Increased energy needs
- Limited access to food

Signs/Symptoms *(Defining Characteristics)*

A typical cluster of subjective and objective signs and symptoms gathered during the nutrition assessment process that provide evidence that a problem exists; quantify the problem and describe its severity.

Nutrition Assessment Category	Potential Indicators of this Nutrition Diagnosis (one or more must be present)
Biochemical Data	
Anthropometric Measurements	• Weight for age less than 5th percentile for infants younger than 12 months • Decreased skinfold thickness and mid-arm muscle circumference (MAMC) • BMI < 18.5 (most adults) • BMI for older adults (over 65 years) < 23 • BMI < 5th percentile (children, 2-19 years)
Physical Exam Findings	• Decreased somatic protein stores, muscle wasting (gluteal and temporal)
Food/Nutrition History	Reports or observations of: • Inadequate intake of food compared to estimated or measured needs

UNDERWEIGHT (NC-3.1)

	• Limited supply of food in home • Dieting, food faddism • Hunger • Refusal to eat • Physical activity greater than recommended amount
Client History	• Malnutrition, vitamin/mineral deficiency • Illness or physical disability • Mental illness, dementia, confusion • Measured resting metabolic rate (RMR) higher than expected and/or estimated RMR • Medications that affect appetite, e.g., stimulants for attention deficit hyperactivity disorder • Athlete, dancer, or gymnast

References:

1. Assessment of nutritional status. In: Kleinman R, ed. *Pediatric Nutrition Handbook,* 5th ed. Chicago, Ill: American Academy of Pediatrics, 2004:407-423.
2. Beck AM, Ovesen LW. At which body mass index and degree of weight loss should hospitalized elderly patients be considered at nutritional risk? *Clin Nutr.* 1998;17:195-198.
3. Blaum CS, Fries BE, Fiatarone MA. Facotors associated with low body mass index and weight loss in nursing home residents. *J Gerontology: Med Sci.* 1995;50A:M162-M168.
4. Position of the American Dietetic Association: Domestic food and nutrition security. *J Am Diet Assoc.* 2002;102:1840-1847.
5. Position of the American Dietetic Association: Addressing world hunger, malnutrition, and food insecurity. *J Am Diet Assoc.* 2003;103:1046-1057.
6. Position of the American Dietetic Association: Nutrition intervention in the treatment of anorexia nervosa, bulimia nervosa, and eating disorder not otherwise specified (EDNOS). *J Am Diet Assoc.* 2001;101:810-819.
7. Schneider SM, Al-Jaouni R, Pivot X, Braulio VB, Rampal P, Hebuerne X. Lack of adaptation to severe malnutrition in elderly patients. *Clin Nutr.* 2002;21(6):499-504.
8. Spear BA. Adolescent growth and development. *J Am Diet Assoc.* 2002 (suppl);102:S23- S29.

INVOLUNTARY WEIGHT LOSS (NC-3.2)

Definition

Decrease in body weight that is not planned or desired

Etiology *(Cause/Contributing Risk Factors)*

Factors gathered during the nutrition assessment process that contribute to the existence or the maintenance of pathophysiological, psychosocial, situational, developmental, cultural, and/or environmental problems:

- Physiologic causes, e.g., increased nutrient needs due to prolonged catabolic illness
- Lack of access to food, e.g., economic constraints, cultural or religious practices, restricting food given to elderly and/or children
- Prolonged hospitalization
- Psychological issues
- Lack of self-feeding ability

Signs/Symptoms *(Defining Characteristics)*

A typical cluster of subjective and objective signs and symptoms gathered during the nutrition assessment process that provide evidence that a problem exists; quantify the problem and describe its severity.

Nutrition Assessment Category	Potential Indicators of this Nutrition Diagnosis (one or more must be present)
Biochemical Data	
Anthropometric Measurements	• Weight loss of 5% within 1 month, 7.5% in 3 months and 10% in 6 months
Physical Examination Findings	• Fever • Increased heart rate • Increased respiratory rate • Loss of subcutaneous fat and muscle stores
Food/Nutrition History	Reports or observations of: • Normal or usual intake in face of illness • Poor intake, change in eating habits, skipped meals • Change in way clothes fit, e.g., becoming looser

INVOLUNTARY WEIGHT LOSS (NC-3.2)

Client History	• Conditions associated with a diagnosis or treatment, e.g., AIDS/HIV, burns, chronic obstructive pulmonary disease, hip/long bone fracture, infection, surgery, trauma, hyperthyroidism (pre-or untreated), some types of cancer or metastatic disease (specify) • Medications associated with weight loss, such as certain antidepressants or cancer chemotherapy

References:

1. Collins N. Protein-energy malnutrition and involuntary weight loss: Nutritional and pharmacologic strategies to enhance wound healing. *Expert Opinion Pharmacother*. 2003;7:1121-1140.
2. Splett PL, Roth-Yousey LL, Vogelzang JL. Medical nutrition therapy for the prevention and treatment of unintentional weight loss in residential healthcare facilities. *J Am Diet Assoc.* 2003; 103:352-362.
3. Wallace JL, Schwartz RS, LaCroix AZ, Uhlmann RF, Pearlman RA. Involuntary weight loss in older patients: incidence and clinical significance. *J Am Geriatr Soc.* 1995;43:329-337.

OVERWEIGHT/OBESITY (NC-3.3)

Definition

Increased adiposity compared to established reference standards or recommendations

Etiology *(Cause/Contributing Risk Factors)*

Factors gathered during the nutrition assessment process that contribute to the existence or the maintenance of pathophysiological, psychosocial, situational, developmental, cultural, and/or environmental problems:

- Decreased energy needs
- Disordered eating pattern
- Excess energy intake
- Food- and nutrition-related knowledge deficit
- Not ready for diet/lifestyle change
- Physical inactivity
- Increased psychological/life stress

Signs/Symptoms *(Defining Characteristics)*

A typical cluster of subjective and objective signs and symptoms gathered during the nutrition assessment process that provide evidence that a problem exists; quantify the problem and describe its severity.

Nutrition Assessment Category	Potential Indicators of this Nutrition Diagnosis (one or more must be present)
Biochemical Data	
Anthropometric Measurements	• BMI above normative standard for age and gender • Waist circumference above normative standard for age and gender • Increased skinfold thickness • Weight for height above normative standard for age and gender
Physical Exam Findings	• Increased body adiposity
Food/Nutrition History	Reports or observations of: • Overconsumption of high-fat and/or calorically-dense food or beverage

OVERWEIGHT/OBESITY (NC-3.3)

	• Large portions of food (portion size greater than twice than recommended) • Excessive energy intake • Infrequent, low-duration and/or low-intensity physical activity • Large amounts of sedentary activities, e.g., TV watching, reading, computer use in both leisure and work/school • Uncertainty regarding nutrition-related recommendations • Inability to apply nutrition-related recommendations • Inability to maintain weight or regain of weight • Unwillingness or disinterest in applying nutrition-related recommendations
Client History	• Conditions associated with a diagnosis or treatment of, e.g., hypothyroidism, metabolic syndrome, eating disorder not otherwise specified, depression • Physical disability or limitation • History of physical, sexual, or emotional abuse • Measured resting metabolic rate (RMR) lower than expected and/or estimated RMR • Medications that impact RMR, e.g., midazolam, propranalol, glipizide

References:

1. Crawford S. Promoting dietary change. *Can J Cardiol.* 1995;11(suppl A):14A-15A.
2. Dickerson RN, Roth-Yousey L. Medication effects on metabolic rate: a systematic review (Part 2). *J Am Diet Assoc.* 2005;105:1002-1009.
3. Dickerson RN, Roth-Yousey L. Medication effects on metabolic rate: a systematic review (Part 1). *J Am Diet Assoc.* 2005;105:835-841.
4. Kumanyika SK, Van Horn L, Bowen D, Perri MG, Rolls BJ, Czajkowski SM, Schron E. Maintenance of dietary behavior change. *Health Psychol.* 2000;19(1 suppl):S42-S56.
5. Position of the American Dietetic Association: Weight management. *J Am Diet Assoc.* 2002;102:1145-1155.
6. Position of the American Dietetic Association: Total diet approach to communicating food and nutrition information. *J Am Diet Assoc* 2002;102:100-108.
7. Position of the American Dietetic Association: The role of dietetics professionals in health promotion and disease prevention. *J Am Diet Assoc.* 2002;102:1680-1687.
8. Position of the American Dietetic Association: Nutrition intervention in the treatment of anorexia nervosa, bulimia nervosa, and eating disorder not otherwise specified (EDNOS). *J Am Diet Assoc.* 2001;101:810-819.
9. Shepherd R. Resistance to changes in diet. *Proc Nutr Soc.* 2002;61:267-272.
10. U.S. Preventive Services Task Force. Behavioral counseling in primary care to promote a healthy diet. *Am J Prev Med.* 2003;24:93-100.

INVOLUNTARY WEIGHT GAIN (NC-3.4)

Definition

Weight gain above that which is desired or planned

Etiology *(Cause/Contributing Risk Factors)*

Factors gathered during the nutrition assessment process that contribute to the existence or the maintenance of pathophysiological, psychosocial, situational, developmental, cultural, and/or environmental problems:

- Illness causing unexpected weight gain because of head trauma, immobility, paralysis or related condition
- Chronic use of medications known to cause weight gain, such as use of certain antidepressants, antipsychotics, corticosteroids, certain HIV medications
- Condition leading to excessive fluid weight gains

Signs/Symptoms *(Defining Characteristics)*

A typical cluster of subjective and objective signs and symptoms gathered during the nutrition assessment process that provide evidence that a problem exists; quantify the problem and describe its severity.

Nutrition Assessment Category	Potential Indicators of this Nutrition Diagnosis (one or more must be present)
Biochemical Data	• Decrease in serum albumin, hyponatremia, elevated fasting serum lipid levels, elevated fasting glucose levels, fluctuating hormone levels
Anthropometric Measurements	• Weight history – noting any increase in weight greater than planned or desired, such as 10% in 6 months • Noticeable change in body fat distribution
Physical Examination Findings	• Fat accumulation—excessive subcutaneous fat stores • Lipodystrophy associated with HIV medications—increase in dorsocervial fat, breast enlargement, increased abdominal girth • Edema • Shortness of breath • Sensitivity to cold, constipation, and hair loss

INVOLUNTARY WEIGHT GAIN (NC-3.4)

Food/Nutrition History	Reports or observations of: • Intake consistent with estimated or measured energy needs • Changes in recent food intake level • Use of alcohol, narcotics • Extreme hunger with or without palpitations, tremor, and sweating • Physical inactivity or change in physical activity level
Client History	• Conditions associated with a diagnosis or treatment of asthma, psychiatric illnesses, rheumatic conditions, HIV/AIDS, Cushing's syndrome, obesity, Prader-Willi syndrome • Fluid administration above requirements • Change in sleep habits, insomnia • Muscle weakness • Fatigue • Medications associated with increased appetite

References:

1. Lichtenstein K, Delaney K, Ward D, Palella F. Clinical factors associated with incidence and prevalence of fat atrophy and accumulation (abstract P64). *Antivir Ther.* 2000; 5:61-62
2. Heath KV, Hogg RS, Chan KJ, Harris M, Montessori V, O'Shaughnessy MV, Montaner JS. Lipodystrophy-associated morphological, cholesterol and triglyceride abnormalities in a population-based HIV/AIDS treatment database. *AIDS.* 2001;15:231-239.
3. Safri S, Grunfeld C. Fat distribution and metabolic changes in patients with HIV infection. *AIDS.* 1999;13:2493-2505.
4. Sattler F. Body habitus changes related to lipodystrophy. *Clin Infect Dis.* 2003;36:S84-S90.

FOOD- AND NUTRITION-RELATED KNOWLEDGE DEFICIT (NB-1.1)

Definition

Incomplete or inaccurate knowledge about food, nutrition, or nutrition-related information and guidelines, e.g., nutrient requirements, consequences of food behaviors, life stage requirements, nutrition recommendations, diseases and conditions, physiological function, or products

Etiology *(Cause/Contributing Risk Factors)*

Factors gathered during the nutrition assessment process that contribute to the existence or the maintenance of pathophysiological, psychosocial, situational, developmental, cultural, and/or environmental problems:

- Harmful beliefs/attitudes about food, nutrition, and nutrition-related topics
- Lack of prior exposure to information
- Language or cultural barrier impacting ability to learn information
- Learning disability, neurological or sensory impairment
- Prior exposure to incompatible information
- Prior exposure to incorrect information
- Unwilling to learn or uninterested in learning information

Signs/Symptoms *(Defining Characteristics)*

A typical cluster of subjective and objective signs and symptoms gathered during the nutrition assessment process that provide evidence that a problem exists; quantify the problem and describe its severity.

Nutrition Assessment Category	Potential Indicators of this Nutrition Diagnosis (one or more must be present)
Biochemical Data	
Anthropometric Measurements	
Physical Exam Findings	

FOOD- AND NUTRITION-RELATED KNOWLEDGE DEFICIT (NB-1.1)

Food/Nutrition History	Observations or reports of: • Verbalizes inaccurate or incomplete information • Provides inaccurate or incomplete written response to questionnaire/written tool, or is unable to read written tool • Demonstrates inability to apply food- and nutrition-related information, e.g., select food based on nutrition therapy or prepare infant feeding as instructed • Relates concerns about previous attempts to learn information • Verbalizes unwillingness to learn or disinterest in learning information
Client History	• Client or caregiver has no prior knowledge of need for food and nutrition-related recommendations • Conditions associated with a diagnosis or treatment of, e.g., mental illness • New medical diagnosis or change in existing diagnosis or condition

References:

1. Crawford S. Promoting dietary change. *Can J Cardiol.* 1995;11(suppl A):14A-15A.
2. Kumanyika SK, Van Horn L, Bowen D, Perri MG, Rolls BJ, Czajkowski SM, Schron E. Maintenance of dietary behavior change. *Health Psychol.* 2000;19(1 suppl):S42-S56.
3. Position of the American Dietetic Association: Weight management. *J Am Diet Assoc.* 2002;102:1145-1155.
4. Position of the American Dietetic Association: Total diet approach to communicating food and nutrition information. *J Am Diet Assoc.* 2002;102:100-108.
5. Position of the American Dietetic Association: The role of dietetics professionals in health promotion and disease prevention. *J Am Diet Assoc.* 2002;102:1680-1687.
6. Shepherd R. Resistance to changes in diet. *Proc Nutr Soc.* 2002;61:267-272.
7. U.S. Preventive Services Task Force. Behavioral counseling in primary care to promote a healthy diet. *Am J Prev Med.* 2003;24:93-100.

HARMFUL BELIEFS/ATTITUDES OR PRACTICES ABOUT FOOD, NUTRITION, AND NUTRITION-RELATED TOPICS (NB-1.2)

Use with caution: Be sensitive to patient concerns.

Definition

Beliefs/attitudes or practices about food, nutrition, and nutrition-related topics that are incompatible with sound nutrition principles, nutrition care or disease/condition (excluding disordered eating patterns and eating disorders)

Etiology (*Cause/Contributing Risk Factors*)

Factors gathered during the nutrition assessment process that contribute to the existence or the maintenance of pathophysiological, psychosocial, situational, developmental, cultural, and/or environmental problems:

- Disbelief in science-based food and nutrition information
- Exposure to incorrect food and nutrition information
- Eating behavior serves a purpose other than nourishment (e.g. Pica)
- Desire for a cure for a chronic disease through the use of alternative therapy

Signs/Symptoms (*Defining Characteristics)*

A typical cluster of subjective and objective signs and symptoms gathered during the nutrition assessment process that provide evidence that a problem exists; quantify the problem and describe its severity.

Nutrition Assessment Category	Potential Indicators of this Nutrition Diagnosis (one or more must be present)
Biochemical Data	
Anthropometric Measurements	
Physical Exam Findings	
Food/Nutrition History	Reports or observations of: • Food fetish, Pica • Food faddism • Intake that reflects an imbalance of nutrients/food groups • Avoidance of foods/food groups (e.g., sugar, wheat, cooked foods)

HARMFUL BELIEFS/ATTITUDES OR PRACTICES ABOUT FOOD, NUTRITION, AND NUTRITION-RELATED TOPICS (NB-1.2)

Client History	• Conditions associated with a diagnosis or treatment, e.g., obesity, diabetes, cancer, cardiovascular disease, mental illness

References:

1. Chapman GE, Beagan B. Women's perspectives on nutrition, health, and breast cancer. *J Nutr Educ Behav*. 2003;35:135-141.
2. Gonzalez VM, Vitousek KM. Feared food in dieting and non-dieting young women: a preliminary validation of the Food Phobia Survey. *Appetite*. 2004;43:155-173.
3. Jowett SL, Seal CJ, Phillips E, Gregory W, Barton JR, Welfare MR. Dietary beliefs of people with ulcerative colitis and their effect on relapse and nutrient intake. *Clin Nutr*. 2004;23:161-170.
4. Madden H, Chamberlain K. Nutritional health messages in women's magazines: a conflicted space for women readers. *J Health Psychology*. 2004;9:583-597.
5. Peters CL, Shelton J, Sharma P. An investigation of factors that influence the consumption of dietary supplements. *Health Mark Psychol*. 2003;21:113-135.
6. Position of the American Dietetic Association: Food and nutrition misinformation. *J Am Diet Assoc*. 2002;102:260-266.
7. Povey R, Wellens B, Conner M. Attitudes towards following meat, vegetarian and vegan diets: an examination of the role of ambivalence. *Appetite*. 2001;37:15-26.
8. Putterman E, Linden W. Appearance versus health: does the reason for dieting affect dieting behavior? *J Behav Med*. 2004;27:185-204.
9. Salminen E, Heikkila S, Poussa T, Lagstrom H, Saario R, Salminen S. Female patients tend to alter their diet following the diagnosis of rheumatoid arthritis and breast cancer. *Prev Med*. 2002;34:529-535.

NOT READY FOR DIET/LIFESTYLE CHANGE (NB-1.3)

Definition

Lack of perceived value of nutrition-related behavior change compared to costs (consequences or effort required to make changes); conflict with personal value system; antecedent to behavior change

Etiology (*Cause/Contributing Risk Factors*)

Factors gathered during the nutrition assessment process that contribute to the existence or the maintenance of pathophysiological, psychosocial, situational, developmental, cultural, and/or environmental problems:

- Harmful beliefs/attitudes about food, nutrition, and nutrition-related topics
- Cognitive deficits or inability to focus on dietary changes
- Lack of social support for implementing changes
- Denial of need to change
- Perception that time, interpersonal, or financial constraints prevent changes
- Unwilling or uninterested in learning information
- Lack of self-efficacy for making change or demoralization from previous failures at change

Signs/Symptoms (*Defining Characteristics*)

A typical cluster of subjective and objective signs and symptoms gathered during the nutrition assessment process that provide evidence that a problem exists; quantify the problem and describe its severity.

Nutrition Assessment Category	Potential Indicators of this Nutrition Diagnosis (one or more must be present)
Biochemical Data	
Anthropometric Measurements	
Physical Exam Findings	• Negative body language, e.g., frowning, lack of eye contact, defensive posture, lack of focus, fidgeting (Note: body language varies by culture.)

NOT READY FOR DIET/LIFESTYLE CHANGE (NB-1.3)

Food/Nutrition History	Reports or observations of: • Denial of need for food- and nutrition-related changes • Inability to understand required changes • Failure to keep appointments/schedule follow-up appointments or engage in counseling • Previous failures to effectively change target behavior • Defensiveness, hostility, or resistance to change • Lack of efficacy to make change or to overcome barriers to change
Client History	• New medical diagnosis, change in existing diagnosis or condition, or chronic non-compliance

References:

1. Crawford S. Promoting dietary change. *Can J Cardiol.* 1995;11:14A-15A.
2. Greene GW, Rossi SR, Rossi JS, Velicer WF, Fava JS, Prochaska JO. Dietary applications of the Stages of Change Model. *J Am Diet Assoc.* 1999;99:673-678.
3. Kumanyika SK, Van Horn L, Bowen D, Perri MG, Rolls BJ, Czajkowski SM, Schron E. Maintenance of dietary behavior change. *Health Psychol.* 2000;19:S42-S56.
4. Prochaska JO, Velicer WF. The Transtheoretical Model of behavior change. *Am J Health Promotion.* 1997;12:38–48.
5. Position of the American Dietetic Association: Total diet approach to communicating food and nutrition information. *J Am Diet Assoc.* 2002;102:100-108.
6. Position of the American Dietetic Association: The role of dietetics professionals in health promotion and disease prevention. *J Am Diet Assoc.* 2002;102:1680-1687.
7. Resnicow K, Jackson A, Wang T, De A, McCarty F, Dudley W, Baronowski T. A motivational interviewing intervention to increase fruit and vegetable intake through black churches: Results of the Eat for Life trial. *Am J Public Health.* 2001;91:1686-1693.
8. Shepherd R. Resistance to changes in diet. *Proc Nutr Soc.* 2002;61:267-272.
9. U.S. Preventive Services Task Force. Behavioral counseling in primary care to promote a healthy diet. *Am J Prev Med.* 2003;24:93-100.

SELF-MONITORING DEFICIT (NB-1.4)

Definition

Lack of data recording to track personal progress

Etiology *(Cause/Contributing Risk Factors)*

Factors gathered during the nutrition assessment process that contribute to the existence or the maintenance of pathophysiological, psychosocial, situational, developmental, cultural, and/or environmental problems:

- Food- and nutrition-related knowledge deficit
- Lack of social support for implementing changes
- Lack of value for behavior change or competing values
- Perception that lack of resources, e.g., time, financial, or social support prevent self-monitoring
- Cultural barrier impacting ability to track personal progress
- Learning disability, neurological, or sensory impairment
- Prior exposure to incompatible information
- Not ready for diet/lifestyle change
- Unwilling or uninterested in tracking progress
- Lack of focus and attention to detail, difficulty with time management and/or organization

Signs/Symptoms *(Defining Characteristics)*

A typical cluster of subjective and objective signs and symptoms gathered during the nutrition assessment process that provide evidence that a problem exists; quantify the problem and describe its severity.

Nutrition Assessment Category	Potential Indicators of this Nutrition Diagnosis (one or more must be present)
Biochemical Data	• Recorded data inconsistent with biochemical data, e.g., dietary intake is not consistent with biochemical data
Anthropometric Measurements	• Recorded data inconsistent with weight status or growth pattern data, e.g., dietary intake is not consistent with weight status or growth pattern
Physical Exam Findings	

SELF-MONITORING DEFICIT (NB-1.4)

Food/Nutrition History	Reports or observations of: • Incomplete self-monitoring records, e.g., glucose, food, fluid intake, weight, physical activity, ostomy output records • Embarrassment or anger regarding need for self-monitoring • Uncertainty of how to complete monitoring records • Uncertainty regarding changes that could/should be made in response to data in self monitoring records • No self management equipment, e.g. no blood glucose monitor, pedometer
Client History	• Diagnoses requiring self-monitoring, e.g., diabetes mellitus, obesity, new ostomy • New medical diagnosis or change in existing diagnosis or condition

References:

1. American Diabetes Association. Tests of glycemia in diabetes. *Diabetes Care.* 2004;27:S91-S93.
2. Baker RC, Kirschenbaum DS. Weight control during the holidays: highly consistent self-monitoring as a potentially useful coping mechanism. *Health Psychol.* 1998;17:367-370.
3. Berkowitz RI, Wadden TA, Tershakovec AM. Behavior therapy and sibutramine for treatment of adolescent obesity. *JAMA.* 2003;289:1805-1812.
4. Crawford S. Promoting dietary change. *Can J Cardiol.* 1995;11(suppl A):14A-15A.
5. Jeffery R, Drewnowski A, Epstein L, Stunkard A, Wilson G, Wing R. Long-term maintenance of weight loss: current status. *Health Psychol.* 2000;19:5-16.
6. Kumanyika SK, Van Horn L, Bowen D, Perri MG, Rolls BJ, Czajkowski SM, Schron E. Maintenance of dietary behavior change. *Health Psychol.* 2000;19(1 suppl):S42-S56.
7. Lichtman SW, Pisaska K, Berman ER, Pestone M, Dowling H, Offenbacher E, Weisel H, Heshka S, Matthews DE, Heymsfield SB. Discrepancy between self-reported and actual caloric intake and exercise in obese subjects. *N Engl J Med* . 1992;327:1893-1898.
8. Wadden, TA. Characteristics of successful weight loss maintainers. In: Allison DB, Pi-Sunyer FX, eds. *Obesity treatment: establishing goals, improving outcomes, and reviewing the research agenda.* New York, NY: Plenum Press;1995:103-111.

DISORDERED EATING PATTERN (NB-1.5)

Definition

Beliefs, attitudes, thoughts and behaviors related to food, eating, and weight management, including classic eating disorders as well as less severe, similar conditions that negatively impact health

Etiology (*Cause/Contributing Risk Factors*)

Factors gathered during the nutrition assessment process that contribute to the existence or the maintenance of pathophysiological, psychosocial, situational, developmental, cultural, and/or environmental problems:

- Obsessive desire to be thin related to familial, societal, biological/genetic, and/or genetic factors
- Weight regulation/preoccupation significantly influences self esteem

Signs/Symptoms (*Defining Characteristics*)

A typical cluster of subjective and objective signs and symptoms gathered during the nutrition assessment process that provide evidence that a problem exists; quantify the problem and describe its severity.

Nutrition Assessment Category	Potential Indicators of this Nutrition Diagnosis (one or more must be present)
Biochemical Data	• Elevated cholesterol, abnormal lipid profiles, hypoglycemia, hypokalemia [anorexia nervosa (AN)] • Hypokalemia and hypochloremic alkalosis [bulimia nervosa (BN)] • Hypotension, bradycardia, low body temperature, hyponatremia, anemia, hypothyroid, leucopenia, elevated BUN (AN) • Urine positive for ketones (AN)
Anthropometric Measurements	• BMI < 17.5, arrested growth and development, failure to gain weight during period of expected growth, weight less than 85% of expected weight (AN) • BMI > 29 [eating disorder not otherwise specified (EDNOS)] • Significant weight fluctuation (BN)

DISORDERED EATING PATTERN (NB-1.5)

Physical Exam Findings	• Severely depleted adipose and somatic protein stores (AN) • Lanugo hair formation on face and trunk, brittle listless hair, cyanosis of hands and feet, and dry skin (AN) • Normal or excess adipose and normal somatic protein stores (BN, EDNOS) • Damaged tooth enamel (BN) • Enlarged parotid glands (BN) • Peripheral edema (BN) • Skeletal muscle loss (AN) • Cardiac arrhythmias (AN, BN) • Irritability, depression (AN, BN) • Inability to concentrate (AN) • Positive Russell's Sign (BN) callous on back of hand from self induced vomiting
Food/Nutrition History	Reports or observations of: • Avoidance of food or calorie-containing beverages (AN, BN) • Fear of foods or dysfunctional thoughts regarding food or food experiences (AN, BN) • Denial of hunger (AN) • Food preoccupation (AN, BN) • Knowledgeable about current diet fad (AN, BN, EDNOS) • Fasting (AN, BN) • Intake of larger quantity of food in a defined time period, a sense of lack of control over eating during the episode (BN, EDNOS) • Excessive physical activity (AN, BN, EDNOS) • Eating much more rapidly than normal, eating until feeling uncomfortably full; consuming large amounts of food when not feeling physically hungry; eating alone because of being embarrassed by how much one is eating; feeling disgusted with oneself, depressed, or very guilty after overeating (EDNOS) • Eats in private (AN, BN) • Irrational thoughts about food's affect on the body (AN, BN, EDNOS) • Pattern of chronic dieting • Weight preoccupation • Excessive reliance on nutrition Terming and preoccupation with nutrient content of foods • Inflexibility with food selection

DISORDERED EATING PATTERN (NB-1.5)

Client History	• Bradycardia (heart rate < 60 beats/min), hypotension (systolic <90 mm Hg), and orthostatic hypotension (AN) • Self-induced vomiting, diarrhea, bloating, constipation and flatulence (BN) • Report of always feeling cold (AN) • Misuse of laxatives, enemas, diuretics, stimulants and/or metabolic enhancers (AN, BN) • Muscle weakness, fatigue, cardiac arrhythmias, dehydration, and electrolyte imbalance (AN, BN) • Diagnosis, e.g., anorexia nervosa, bulimia nervosa, binge eating, eating disorder not otherwise specified, amenorrhea • History of mood and anxiety disorders (e.g., depression, obsessive compulsive disorder), personality disorders, substance abuse disorders • Family history of ED, depression, OCD, anxiety disorders (AN, BN) • Avoidance of social events where food is served

References:

1. Anderson GH, Kennedy SH, eds. *The Biology of Feast and Famine*. New York: Academic Press; 1992.
2. American Psychiatric Association. *Diagnostic and Statistical Manual for Mental Disorders (Fourth Edition, Text Revision)*. Washington, DC: APA Press; 2000.
3. American Psychiatric Association. Practice guidelines for the treatment of patients with eating disorders. *Am J Psychiatry*. 2000;157 (suppl):1-39.
4. Cooke RA, Chambers JB. Anorexia nervosa and the heart. *Br J Hosp Med*. 1995;54:313-317.
5. Fisher M. Medical complications of anorexia and bulimia nervosa. *Adol Med*. 1992;3:481-502.
6. Gralen SJ, Levin MP, Smolak L et al. Dieting and disordered eating during early and middle adolescents: Do the influences remain the same? *Int J Eat Disord*. 1990;9:501-512.
7. Harris JP, Kriepe RE, Rossback CN. QT prolongation by isoproterenol in anorexia nervosa. *J Adol Health*. 1993;14:390-393.
8. Kaplan AS, Garfunkel PE, eds. *Medical Issues and the Eating Disorders: The Interface*. New York,NY: Brunner/Manzel Publishers; 1993.
9. Keys A, Brozek J, Henschel A, Mickelson O, Taylor HL. *The Biology of Human Starvation, 2nd vol*. Minneapolis, Minn: University of Minnesota Press; 1950.
10. Kirkley BG. Bulimia: clinical characteristics, development, and etiology. *J Am Diet Assoc*. 1986;86:468-475.
11. Kreipe RE, Uphoff M. Treatment and outcome of adolescents with anorexia nervosa. *Adolesc Med*.1992;16:519-540.
12. Kreipe RE, Birndorf DO. Eating disorders in adolescents and young adults. *Med Clin N Am*. 2000;84(4):1027-1049.
13. Mordasini R, Klose G, Greter H. Secondary type II hyperlipoproteinemia in patients with anorexia nervosa. *Metabolism*. 1978;27:71-79.
14. Position of the American Dietetic Association: Nutrition intervention in the treatment of anorexia nervosa, bulimia nervosa, and eating disorder not otherwise specified (EDNOS). *J Am Diet Assoc*. 2001;101:810-819.
16. Rock C, Yager J. Nutrition and eating disorders: a primer for clinicians. *Int J Eat Disord*. 1987;6:267-280.
17. Rock CL. Nutritional and medical assessment and management of eating disorders. *Nutr Clin Care*. 1999;2:332-343.
18. Schebendach J, Reichert-Anderson P. Nutrition in Eating Disorders. In: Mahan K, Escott-Stump S, eds. *Kraus's Nutrition and Diet Therapy*. New York, NY: McGraw- Hill; 2000.
19. Silber T. Anorexia nervosa: Morbidity and mortality. *Peiatr Ann*. 1984;13:851-859.
20. Swenne I. Heart risk associated with weight loss in anorexia nervosa and eating disorders: electrocardiographic changes during the early phase of refeeding. *Acta Paediatr*. 2000;89:447-452.
21. Turner JM, Bulsara MK, McDermott BM, Byrne GC, Prince RL, Forbes DA. Predictors of low bone density in young adolescent females with anorexia nervosa and other dieting disorders. *Int J Eat Disord*. 2001;30:245-251.

LIMITED ADHERENCE TO NUTRITION-RELATED RECOMMENDATIONS (NB-1.6)

Definition

Lack of nutrition-related changes as per intervention agreed upon by client or population

Etiology *(Cause/Contributing Risk Factors)*

Factors gathered during the nutrition assessment process that contribute to the existence or the maintenance of pathophysiological, psychosocial, situational, developmental, cultural, and/or environmental problems:

- Lack of social support for implementing changes
- Lack of value for behavior change or competing values
- Perception that time or financial constraints prevent changes
- Previous lack of success in making health-related changes
- Poor understanding of how and why to make changes
- Unwilling to applyor uninterested in applying information

Signs/Symptoms *(Defining Characteristics)*

A typical cluster of subjective and objective signs and symptoms gathered during the nutrition assessment process that provide evidence that a problem exists; quantify the problem and describe its severity.

Nutrition Assessment Category	**Potential Indicators of this Nutrition Diagnosis (one or more must be present)**
Biochemical Data	• Expected laboratory outcomes are not achieved
Anthropometric Measurements	• Expected anthropometric outcomes are not achieved
Physical Exam Findings	• Negative body language, e.g., frowning, lack of eye contact, fidgeting (Note: body language varies by culture)

LIMITED ADHERENCE TO NUTRITION-RELATED RECOMMENDATIONS (NB-1.6)

Food/Nutrition History	Reports or observations of: • Expected food/nutrition-related outcomes are not achieved • Inability to recall agreed upon changes • Failure to complete any agreed upon homework • Lack of compliance or inconsistent compliance with plan • Failure to keep appointments or schedule follow-up appointments • Lack of appreciation of the importance of making recommended nutrition-related changes • Uncertainty as to how to consistently apply food/nutrition information
Client History	

References:

1. Crawford S. Promoting dietary change. *Can J Cardiol.* 1995;11(suppl A):14A-15A.
2. Kumanyika SK, Van Horn L, Bowen D, Perri MG, Rolls BJ, Czajkowski SM, Schron E. Maintenance of dietary behavior change. *Health Psychol.* 2000;19(1 suppl):S42-S56.
3. Position of the American Dietetic Association: Total diet approach to communicating food and nutrition information. *J Am Diet Assoc.* 2002;102:100-108.
4. Shepherd R. Resistance to changes in diet. *Proc Nutr Soc.* 2002;61:267-272.
5. U.S. Preventive Services Task Force. Behavioral counseling in primary care to promote a healthy diet. *Am J Prev Med.* 2003;24:93-100.

UNDESIRABLE FOOD CHOICES (NB-1.7)

Definition

Food and/or beverage choices that are inconsistent with US Recommended Dietary Intake, US Dietary Guidelines, or with the My Pyramid or with targets defined in the nutrition prescription or nutrition care process

Etiology (*Cause/Contributing Risk Factors*)

Factors gathered during the nutrition assessment process that contribute to the existence or the maintenance of pathophysiological, psychosocial, situational, developmental, cultural, and/or environmental problems:

- Lack of prior exposure to or misunderstanding of information
- Language, religious, or cultural barriers affecting ability to apply information
- Learning disabilities, neurological or sensory impairment
- High level of fatigue or other side effect of therapy
- Inadequate access to recommended foods
- Perception that financial constraints prevent selection of food choices consistent with recommendations
- Food allergies and aversions impeding food choices consistent with guidelines
- Lacks motivation and/or readiness to apply or support systems change
- Unwilling or uninterested in learning information
- Psychological limitations

Signs/Symptoms (*Defining Characteristics*)

A typical cluster of subjective and objective signs and symptoms gathered during the nutrition assessment process that provide evidence that a problem exists; quantify the problem and describe its severity.

Nutrition Assessment Category	Potential Indicators of this Nutrition Diagnosis (one or more must be present)
Biochemical Data	• Elevated lipid panel
Anthropometric Measurements	
Physical Exam Findings	• Findings consistent with vitamin/mineral deficiency or excess

UNDESIRABLE FOOD CHOICES (NB-1.7)

Food/Nutrition History	Reports or observations of: • Intake inconsistent with US Dietary Guidelines or My Pyramid (e.g., omission of entire nutrient groups, disproportionate intake such as juice for young children]) • Inaccurate or incomplete understanding of the guidelines • Inability to apply guideline information • Inability (e.g. access) or unwillingness to select, or disinterest in selecting food consistent with the guidelines
Client History	• Conditions associated with a diagnosis or treatment, e.g., mental illness

References:

1. Birch LL, Fisher JA. Appetite and eating behavior in children. *Pediatr Clin North Am.* 1995:42;931-953.
2. Butte N, Cobb K, Dwyer J, Graney L, Heird W, Richard K. The start healthy feeding guidelines for infants and toddlers. *J Am Diet Assoc.* 2004;104:442-454.
3. Position of the American Dietetic Association: Weight management. *J Am Diet Assoc.* 2002;102:1145-1155.
4. Dolecek TA, Stamlee J, Caggiula AW, Tillotson JL, Buzzard IM. Methods of dietary and nutritional assessment and intervention and other methods in the multiple risk factor intervention trial. *Am J Clin Nutr.* 1997;65(suppl):196S-210S.
5. Epstein LH, Gordy CC, Raynor HA, Beddome M, Kilanowski CK, Paluch R. Increasing fruit and vegetable intake and decreasing fat and sugar intake in families at risk for childhood obesity. *Obesity Res.* 2001;9:171-178.
6. Freeland-Graves J, Nitzke S. Total diet approach to communicating food and nutrition information. *J Am Diet Assoc.* 2002;102:100-108.
7. French SA. Pricing effects on food choices. *J Nutr.* 2003;133 (suppl):841S-843S.
8. Glens K, Basil M, Mariachi E, Goldberg J, Snyder D. Why Americans eat what they do: taste, nutrition, cost, convenience and weight control concerns as influences on food consumption. *J Am Diet Assoc.* 1998;98:1118-1126.
9. Hampl JS, Anderson JV, Mullis R. The role of dietetics professionals in health promotion and disease prevention. *J Am Diet Assoc.* 2002;102:1680-1687.
10. Lin SH, Guthrie J, Frazao E. American children's' diets are not making the grade. *Food Rev.* 2001;24:8-17.
11. Satter E. Feeding dynamics: helping children to eat well. *J Pediatr Healthcare.* 1995;9:178-184.
12. Story M, Holt K, Sofka D, eds. *Bright Futures in Practice: Nutrition, 2nd ed.* Arlington, Va: National Center for Education in Maternal Child Health; 2002.
13. Pelto GH, Levitt E, Thairu L. Improving feeding practices, current patterns, common constraints and the design of interventions. *Food Nutr Bull.* 2003;24:45-82.

PHYSICAL INACTIVITY (NB-2.1)

Definition

Low level of activity/sedentary behavior to the extent that it reduces energy expenditure and impacts health

Etiology (*Cause/Contributing Risk Factors*)

Factors gathered during the nutrition assessment process that contribute to the existence or the maintenance of pathophysiological, psychosocial, situational, developmental, cultural, and/or environmental problems:

- Financial constraints that may prevent sufficient level of activity
- Harmful beliefs/attitudes about physical activity
- Injury or lifestyle change that reduces physical activity or activities of daily living
- Lack of prior education about need for physical activity or how to incorporate exercise, e.g., physical disability, arthritis
- Lack of role models, e.g., for children
- Lack of social support and/or environmental space or equipment
- Lack of safe environment for physical activity
- Lack of value or competing values for behavior change
- Time constraints

Signs/Symptoms (*Defining Characteristics*)

A typical cluster of subjective and objective signs and symptoms gathered during the nutrition assessment process that provide evidence that a problem exists; quantify the problem and describe its severity.

Nutrition Assessment Category	Potential Indicators of this Nutrition Diagnosis (one or more must be present)
Biochemical Data	
Anthropometric Measurements	
Physical Exam Findings	

PHYSICAL INACTIVITY (NB-2.1)

Food/Nutrition History	Reports or observations of: • Infrequent, low-duration and/or low-intensity physical activity • Large amounts of sedentary activities, e.g., TV watching, reading, computer use in both leisure and work/school • Barriers to physical activity, e.g., time constraints, availability of a safe environment for exercise
Client History	• Low cardio-respiratory fitness and/or low muscle strength • Medical diagnoses that may be associated with or result in decreased activity, e.g., arthritis, chronic fatigue syndrome, morbid obesity, knee surgery • Medications that cause somnolence and decreased cognition • Psychological diagnosis, e.g., depression, anxiety disorders

References:

1. Position of the American Dietetic Association: Weight management. *J Am Diet Assoc.* 2002;102:1145-1155.
2. Position of the American Dietetic Association: Total diet approach to communicating food and nutrition information. *J Am Diet Assoc.* 2002;102:100-108.
3. Position of the American Dietetic Association: The role of dietetics professionals in health promotion and disease prevention. *J Am Diet Assoc.* 2002;102:1680-1687.

EXCESSIVE EXERCISE (NB-2.2)

Definition

An amount of exercise that exceeds that which is necessary to improve health and/or athletic performance

Etiology *(Cause/Contributing Risk Factors)*

Factors gathered during the nutrition assessment process that contribute to the existence or the maintenance of pathophysiological, psychosocial, situational, developmental, cultural, and/or environmental problems:

- Disordered eating
- Irrational beliefs/attitudes about food, nutrition, and fitness
- "Addictive" behaviors/personality

Signs/Symptoms *(Defining Characteristics)*

A typical cluster of subjective and objective signs and symptoms gathered during the nutrition assessment process that provide evidence that a problem exists; quantify the problem and describe its severity.

Nutrition Assessment Category	Potential Indicators of this Nutrition Diagnosis (one or more must be present)
Biochemical Data	• Elevated liver enzymes, e.g., LDH, SGOT • Altered micronutrient status, e.g., decreased serum ferritin, zinc, and IGF-binding protein • Increased hematocrit • Suppressed immune function • Possibly elevated cortisol levels
Anthropometric Measurements	• Weight loss, arrested growth and development, failure to gain weight during period of expected growth (related usually to disordered eating)
Physical Exam Findings	• Depleted adipose and somatic protein stores (related usually to disordered eating) • Frequent and/or prolonged injuries and/or illnesses • Chronic fatigue • Chronic muscle soreness

EXCESSIVE EXERCISE (NB-2.2)

Food/Nutrition History	Reports or observations of: • Continued/repeated high levels of exercise exceeding levels necessary to improve health and/or athletic performance • Exercise daily without rest/rehabilitation days • Exercise while injured/sick • Forsaking family, job, social responsibilities to exercise
Client History	• Conditions associated with a diagnosis or treatment of, e.g., anorexia nervosa, bulimia nervosa, binge eating, eating disorder not otherwise specified, amenorrhea • Evidence of addictive, obsessive, or compulsive tendencies

References:

1. Aissa-Benhaddad A, Bouix D, Khaled S, Micallef JP, Mercier J, Bringer J, Brun JF. Early hemorheologic aspects of overtraining in elite athletes. *Clin Hemorheol Microcirc.* 1999;20:117-125.
2. American Psychiatric Association. *Diagnostic and Statistical Manual of Mental Disorders.* 4th ed. Washington, DC: American Psychiatric Association; 2000.
3. Davis C, Brewer H, Ratusny D. Behavioral frequency and psychological commitment: necessary concepts in the study of excessive exercising. *J Behav Med.* 1993;16:611-628
4. Davis C, Claridge G. The eating disorder as addiction: a psychobiological perspective. *Addict Behav.* 1998;23:463-475.
5. Davis C, Kennedy SH, Ravelski E, Dionne M. The role of physical activity in the development and maintenance of eating disorders. *Psychol Med.* 1994;24:957-967.
6. Klein DA, Bennett AS, Schebendach J, Foltin RW, Devlin MJ, Walsh BT. Exercise "addiction" in anorexia nervosa: model development and pilot data. *CNS Spectr.* 2004;9:531-537.
7. Lakier-Smith L. Overtraining, excessive exercise, and altered immunity: this a helper-1 vs helper-2 lymphocyte response? *Sports Med.* 2003;33:347-364.
8. Position of the American Dietetic Association: Nutrition intervention in the treatment of anorexia nervosa, bulimia nervosa, and eating disorder not otherwise specified (EDNOS). *J Am Diet Assoc.* 2001;101:810-819.
9. Shephard RJ, Shek PN. Acute and chronic over-exertion: do depressed immune responses provide useful markers? *Int J Sports Med.* 1998;19:159-171.
10. Smith LL. Tissue trauma: the underlying cause of overtraining syndrome? *J Strength Cond Res.* 2004;18:185-193.
11. Urhausen A, Kindermann W. Diagnosis of overtraining: what tools do we have. *Sports Med.* 2002;32:95-102.

INABILITY OR LACK OF DESIRE TO MANAGE SELF-CARE (NB-2.3)

Definition

Lack of capacity or unwillingness to implement methods to support healthful food- and nutrition-related behavior

Etiology (*Cause/Contributing Risk Factors*)

Factors gathered during the nutrition assessment process that contribute to the existence or the maintenance of pathophysiological, psychosocial, situational, developmental, cultural, and/or environmental problems:

- Food- and nutrition-related knowledge deficit
- Lack of caretaker or social support for implementing changes
- Lack of developmental readiness to perform self management tasks, e.g. pediatrics
- Lack of value or competing values for behavior change
- Perception that lack of resources (time, financial, support persons) prevent self care
- Cultural beliefs and practices
- Learning disability, neurological or sensory impairment
- Prior exposure to incompatible information
- Not ready for diet/lifestyle change
- Unwilling or uninterested in learning/applying information
- No self-management tools or decision guides

Signs/Symptoms (*Defining Characteristics*)

A typical cluster of subjective and objective signs and symptoms gathered during the nutrition assessment process that provide evidence that a problem exists; quantify the problem and describe its severity.

Nutrition Assessment Category	Potential Indicators of this Nutrition Diagnosis (one or more must be present)
Biochemical Data	
Anthropometric Measurements	
Physical Exam Findings	

INABILITY OR LACK OF DESIRE TO MANAGE SELF-CARE (NB-2.3)

Food/Nutrition History	Reports or observations of: • Inability to interpret data or self-management tools • Embarrassment or anger regarding need for self-monitoring • Uncertainty regarding changes that could/should be made in response to data in self-monitoring records
Client History	• Diagnoses that are associated with self management, e.g., diabetes mellitus, obesity, cardiovascular disease, renal or liver disease • Conditions associated with a diagnosis or treatment, e.g., cognitive or emotional impairment • New medical diagnosis or change in existing diagnosis or condition

References:

1. Position of the American Dietetic Association: Providing nutrition services for infants, children, and adults with developmental disabilities and special health care needs. *J Am Diet Assoc.* 2004;104:97-107.
2. Crawford S. Promoting dietary change. *Can J Cardiol.* 1995;11(suppl A):14A-15A.
3. Falk LW, Bisogni CA, Sobal J. Diet change processes of participants in an intensive heart program. *J Nutr Educ.* 2000;32:240-250.
4. Glasgow RE, Hampson SE, Strycker LA, Ruggiero L. Personal-model beliefs and social-environmental barriers related to diabetes self-management. *Diabetes Care.* 1997;20:556-561.
5. Keenan DP, AbuSabha R, Sigman-Grant M, Achterberg C, Ruffing J. Factors perceived to influence dietary fat reduction behaviors. *J Nutr Educ.*1999;31:134-144.
6. Kumanyika SK, Van Horn L, Bowen D, Perri MG, Rolls BJ, Czajkowski SM, Schron E. Maintenance of dietary behavior change. *Health Psychol.* 2000;19(1 suppl):S42-S56.
7. Sporny, LA, Contento IR. Stages of change in dietary fat reduction: Social psychological correlates. *J Nutr Educ.* 1995;27:191.

IMPAIRED ABILITY TO PREPARE FOODS/MEALS (NB-2.4)

Definition

Cognitive or physical impairment that prevents preparation of foods/meals

Etiology (*Cause/Contributing Risk Factors*)

Factors gathered during the nutrition assessment process that contribute to the existence or the maintenance of pathophysiological, psychosocial, situational, developmental, cultural, and/or environmental problems:

- Learning disability, neurological or sensory impairment
- Loss of mental or cognitive ability, e.g., dementia
- Physical disability
- High level of fatigue or other side effect of therapy

Signs/Symptoms (*Defining Characteristics*)

A typical cluster of subjective and objective signs and symptoms gathered during the nutrition assessment process that provide evidence that a problem exists; quantify the problem and describe its severity.

Nutrition Assessment Category	Potential Indicators of this Nutrition Diagnosis (one or more must be present)
Biochemical Data	
Anthropometric Measurements	
Physical Exam Findings	
Food/Nutrition History	Observations or reports of: • Decreased overall intake • Excessive consumption of convenience foods, pre-prepared meals, and foods prepared away from home resulting in an inability to adhere to nutrition prescription • Uncertainty regarding appropriate foods to prepare based upon nutrition prescription • Inability to purchase and transport foods to one's home
Client History	• Conditions associated with a diagnosis or treatment, e.g., cognitive impairment, cerebral palsy, paraplegia, sight impairment, rigorous therapy regimen, recent surgery

IMPAIRED ABILITY TO PREPARE FOODS/MEALS (NB-2.4)

References:

1. Andren E, Grimby G. Activity limitations in personal, domestic and vocational tasks: a study of adults with inborn and early acquired mobility disorders. *Disabil Rehabil.* 2004;26:262-271.
2. Andren E, Grimby G. Dependence in daily activities and life satisfaction in adult subjects with cerebral palsy or spina bifida: a follow-up study. *Disabil Rehabil.* 2004;26:528-536.
3. Fortin S, Godbout L, Braun CM. Cognitive structure of executive deficits in frontally lesioned head trauma patients performing activities of daily living. *Cortex.* 2003;39:273-291.
4. Godbout L, Doucet C, Fiola M. The scripting of activities of daily living in normal aging: anticipation and shifting deficits with preservation of sequencing. *Brain Cogn.* 2000;43:220-224.
5. Position of the American Dietetic Association: Providing nutrition services for infants, children, and adults with developmental disabilities and special health care needs. *J Am Diet Assoc.* 2004;104:97-107.
6. Position of the American Dietetic Association: Domestic food and nutrition security. *J Am Diet Assoc.* 2002;102:1840-1847.
7. Position of the American Dietetic Association: Addressing world hunger, malnutrition, and food insecurity. *J Am Diet Assoc.* 2003;103:1046-1057.
8. Sandstrom K, Alinder J, Oberg B. Descriptions of functioning and health and relations to a gross motor classification in adults with cerebral palsy. *Disabil Rehabil.* 2004;26:1023-1031.

POOR NUTRITION QUALITY OF LIFE (NQOL) (NB-2.5)

Definition

Diminished NQOL scores related to food impact, self image, psychological factors, social/interpersonal factors, physical factors, or self-efficacy

Etiology *(Cause/Contributing Risk Factors)*

Factors gathered during the nutrition assessment process that contribute to the existence or the maintenance of pathophysiological, psychosocial, situational, developmental, cultural, and/or environmental problems.

- Food- and nutrition knowledge-related deficit
- Not ready for diet/lifestyle change
- Negative impact of current or previous medical nutrition therapy (MNT)
- Food or activity behavior-related difficulty
- Poor self-efficacy
- Altered body image
- Food insecurity
- Lack of social support for implementing changes

Signs/Symptoms *(Defining Characteristics)*

A typical cluster of subjective and objective signs and symptoms gathered during the nutrition assessment process that provide evidence that a problem exists; quantify the problem and describe its severity.

Nutrition Assessment Category	Potential Indicators of this Nutrition Diagnosis (one or more must be present)
Biochemical Data	
Anthropometric Measurements	
Physical Exam Findings	

POOR NUTRITION QUALITY OF LIFE (NQOL) (NB-2.5)

Food/Nutrition History	Reports or observations of: • Unfavorable NQOL rating • Frustration or dissatisfaction with MNT recommendations • Inaccurate or incomplete information related to MNT recommendations • Inability to change food- or activity-related behavior • Concerns about previous attempts to learn information • Unwillingness or disinterest in learning information
Client History	• New medical diagnosis or change in existing diagnosis or condition • Recent other lifestyle or life changes, e.g., quit smoking, initiated exercise, work change, home relocation

References:

1. Barr JT, Schumacher GE. The need for a nutrition-related quality-of-life measure. *J Am Diet Assoc.* 2003;103:177-180.
2. Barr JT, Schumacher GE. Using focus groups to determine what constitutes quality of life in clients receiving medical nutrition therapy: First steps in the development of a nutrition quality-of-life survey. *J Am Diet Assoc.* 2003;103:844-851.

SELF-FEEDING DIFFICULTY (NB-2.6)

Definition

Impaired actions to place food or beverages in mouth

Etiology *(Cause/Contributing Risk Factors)*

Factors gathered during the nutrition assessment process that contribute to the existence or the maintenance of pathophysiological, psychosocial, situational, developmental, cultural, and/or environmental problems:

- Inability to grasp cups and utensils for self-feeding
- Inability to support and/or control head and neck
- Lack of coordination of hand to mouth
- Limited physical strength or range of motion
- Inability to bend elbow or wrist
- Inability to sit with hips square and back straight
- Limited access to foods conducive for self-feeding
- Limited vision
- Reluctance or avoidance of self feeding

Signs/Symptoms *(Defining Characteristics)*

A typical cluster of subjective and objective signs and symptoms gathered during the nutrition assessment process that provide evidence that a problem exists; quantify the problem and describe its severity.

Nutrition Assessment Category	Potential Indicators of this Nutrition Diagnosis (one or more must be present)
Biochemical Data	
Anthropometric Measurements	
Physical Exam Findings	• Dry mucous membranes, hoarse or wet voice, tongue extrusion

SELF-FEEDING DIFFICULTY (NB-2.6)

Food/Nutrition History	Reports or observations of: • Being provided with foods that may not be conducive to self-feeding, e.g., peas, broth-type soups • Poor lip closure, drooling • Dropping of cups, utensils • Emotional distress, anxiety, or frustration surrounding mealtimes • Failure to recognize foods • Forgets to eat • Inappropriate use of food • Refusal to eat or chew • Dropping of food from utensil (splashing and spilling of food) on repeated attempts to feed • Utensil biting
Client History	• Conditions associated with a diagnosis or treatment of, e.g., neurological disorders, Parkinson's disease, Alzheimer's disease, Tardive dyskinesia, multiple sclerosis, stroke, paralysis, developmental delay • Physical limitations, e.g., fractured arms, traction, contractures • Surgery requiring recumbent position • Dementia/organic brain syndrome • Dysphagia • Weight loss • Shortness of breath • Tremors

References:

1. Consultant Dietitians in Healthcare Facilities. *Dining Skills Supplement: Practical Interventions for Caregivers of Eating Disabled Older Adults.* Pensacola, Fla: American Dietetic Association; 1992.
2. Morley JE. Anorexia of aging: physiological and pathologic. *Am J Clin Nutr.* 1997;66:760-773.
3. Position of the American Dietetic Association: Providing nutrition services for infants, children, and adults with developmental disabilities and special health care needs. *J Am Diet Assoc.* 2004;104:97-107.
4. Sandman P, Norberg A, Adolfsson R, Eriksson S, Nystrom L. Prevalence and characteristics of persons with dependency on feeding at institutions. *Scand J Caring Sci.* 1990;4:121-127.
5. Siebens H, Trupe E, Siebens A, Cooke F, Anshen S, Hanauer R, Oster G. Correlates and consequences of feeding dependency. *J Am Geriatr Soc.* 1986;34:192-198.
6. Vellas B, Fitten LJ, eds. *Research and Practice in Alzheimer's Disease.* New York, NY: Springer Publishing Company; 1998.

INTAKE OF UNSAFE FOOD (NB-3.1)

Definition

Intake of food and/or fluids intentionally or unintentionally contaminated with toxins, poisonous products, infectious agents, microbial agents, additives, allergens, and/or agents of bioterrorism

Etiology *(Cause/Contributing Risk Factors)*

Factors gathered during the nutrition assessment process that contribute to the existence or the maintenance of pathophysiological, psychosocial, situational, developmental, cultural, and/or environmental problems:

- Lack of knowledge about potentially unsafe food
- Lack of knowledge about proper food/feeding, storage and preparation, e.g., infant and enteral formula, or breast milk
- Exposure to contaminated water or food, e.g., community outbreak of illness documented by surveillance and/or response agency
- Mental illness, confusion or altered awareness
- Inadequate food storage equipment/facilities, e.g., refrigerator
- Inadequate safe food supply, e.g., inadequate access to markets with safe, uncontaminated food

Signs/Symptoms *(Defining Characteristics)*

A typical cluster of subjective and objective signs and symptoms gathered during the nutrition assessment process that provide evidence that a problem exists; quantify the problem and describe its severity.

Nutrition Assessment Category	Potential Indicators of this Nutrition Diagnosis (one or more must be present)
Biochemical Data	• Positive stool culture for infectious causes, such as listeria, salmonella, hepatitis A, *E. coli*, *cyclospora* • Toxicology reports for drugs, medicinals, poisons in blood or food samples
Anthropometric Measurements	
Physical Examination Findings	• Evidence of dehydration, e.g., dry mucous membranes, damaged tissues

INTAKE OF UNSAFE FOOD (NB-3.1)

Food/Nutrition History	Observations/reports of intake of potential unsafe foods (e.g., pregnant and lactating women): • Mercury content of fish and in non-food items • Raw eggs, unpasteurized milk products, soft cheeses, undercooked meats (infants, children, immunocompromised persons, pregnant and lactating women, and elderly) • Wild plants, berries, and mushrooms Observations/reports of unsafe food/feeding or storage and preparation practices (enteral and infant formula, or breast milk)
Client History	• Conditions associated with a diagnosis or treatment of, e.g., food borne illness, such as, bacterial, viral, and parasitic infection, mental illness, dementia • Poisoning by drugs, medicinals, or biological substances • Poisoning from poisonous food stuffs or poisonous plants • Diarrhea, cramping, bloating, fever, nausea, vomiting, vision problems, chills, dizziness, headache • Cardiac, neurologic, respiratory changes

References:

1. Centers for Disease Control and Prevention. Diagnosis and Management of Foodborne Illness: A Primer for Physicians. Available at: www.cdc.gov/mmwr/preview/mmwrhtml/rr5304a1.htm. Accessed July 2, 2004.
2. Food Safety and Inspection Service. The Fight BAC Survey Tool and Data Entry Tool. Available at: www.fsis.usda.gov/OA/fses/bac_datatool.htm. Accessed July 2, 2004.
3. Gerald BL, Perkin JE. Food and water safety. *J Am Diet Assoc.* 2003;103:1203-1218.
4. Partnership for Food Safety Education. Four steps. Available at: http://www.fightbac.org/foursteps.cfm?section=4. Accessed July 2, 2004.

LIMITED ACCESS TO FOOD (NB-3.2)

Definition

Diminished ability to acquire food from sources (e.g., shopping, gardening, meal delivery), due to financial constraints, physical impairment, caregiver support, or unsafe living conditions (e.g. crime hinders travel to grocery store). Limitation to food because of concerns about weight or aging.

Etiology (*Cause/Contributing Risk Factors*)

Factors gathered during the nutrition assessment process that contribute to the existence or the maintenance of pathophysiological, psychosocial, situational, developmental, cultural, and/or environmental problems:

- Caregiver intentionally or unintentionally not providing access to food, e.g., unmet needs for food or eating assistance, abuse/neglect
- Community and geographical constraints for shopping and transportation
- Lack of financial resources or lack of access to financial resources to purchase sufficient food
- Limited or absent community supplemental food programs, e.g., food pantry, shelter
- Failure to participate in food programs such as WIC, National School Lunch Program, food stamps
- Physical or psychological limitations that diminish ability to shop, e.g., walking, sight, mental/emotional health

Signs/Symptoms (*Defining Characteristics*)

A typical cluster of subjective and objective signs and symptoms gathered during the nutrition assessment process that provide evidence that a problem exists; quantify the problem and describe its severity.

Nutrition Assessment Category	Potential Indicators of this Nutrition Diagnosis (one or more must be present)
Biochemical Data	• Indicators of macronutrient or vitamin/mineral status
Anthropometric Measurements	• Growth failure, based on National Center for Health Statistics (NCHS) growth standards • Underweight (BMI < 18.5)
Physical Exam Findings	• Findings consistent with vitamin or mineral deficiency

LIMITED ACCESS TO FOOD (NB-3.2)

Food/Nutrition History	Reports or observations of: • Food faddism • Belief that aging can be slowed by dietary limitations and extreme exercise • Hunger • Inadequate intake of food and/or specific nutrients • Limited supply of food in home • Limited variety of foods
Client History	• Malnutrition, vitamin or mineral deficiency • Illness or physical disability • Conditions associated with a diagnosis or treatment, e.g., mental illness, dementia • Lack of suitable support systems

References:

1. Position of the American Dietetic Association: Domestic food and nutrition security. *J Am Diet Assoc.* 2002;102:1840-1847.
2. Position of the American Dietetic Association: Addressing world hunger, malnutrition, and food insecurity. *J Am Diet Assoc.* 2003;103:1046-1057.

SUBJECT: NUTRITION CONTROLLED VOCABULARY/TERMINOLOGY MAINTENANCE/REVIEW

AMERICAN DIETETIC ASSOCIATION
120 South Riverside Plaza Suite 2000
CHICAGO, ILLINOIS 60606-6995

Effective Date: April 2005
Revision Date: June 2006
Review Date:

PURPOSE:
This policy establishes the process followed by the Nutrition Care Process/Standardized Language (NCP/SL) Committee to maintain a current Nutrition Care Process and list of nutrition controlled vocabulary terminology that document the Nutrition Care Process.

STRUCTURE:
The NCP/SL Committee is a joint House of Delegates and Board of Directors Committee and provides semi-annual reports to both bodies.

PROCEDURES:
The NCP/SL Committee accepts proposals for modification or additions to the Nutrition Diagnostic Terminology as follows:

1. Any individual ADA member or Dietetic Practice Group can submit proposals for modification or additions by completing the attached two documents:
    a. Proposed Nutrition Diagnostic Terminology Modification/Addition letter
    b. Reference worksheet for proposed modification/addition
2. The NCP/SL will review the submissions at their routine face-to-face meetings or teleconferences to establish the following:
    a. Is the term already represented by an existing term?
        i. If so the new term can be added as a synonym for the existing term or replace the existing term.
        ii. If not, then the term can be considered for addition to the list of terms as long as it meets the need for describing elements of dietetic practice in the context of the nutrition care process.
    b. Does the term overlap with an existing term, but add new elements?
        i. If yes, then the existing term can be modified to include the new elements or the proposed term can be clarified to be distinctly different from the existing term through a dialogue with the proposal submitter.
        ii. If no, then consider adding new term.
    c. Is the term distinct and separate from all existing terms?
        i. If yes, then ensure that the term is in the context of dietetic practice within the Nutrition Care Process and consider adding to list of terms.
        ii. If no, then work with proposal submitter to discuss how to integrate into existing terms or create a separate term.
3. The NCP/SL Committee will prepare a summary of comments and one representative of the NCP/SL will confer with the proposal submitter after the initial discussion to answer questions and discuss the initial input from the NCP/SL Committee. If the proposal

questions and discuss the initial input from the NCP/SL Committee. If the proposal submitter is not satisfied with the direction proposed by the NCP/SL Committee, then they will be invited to submit additional documentation and have time on the next teleconference/meeting agenda to personally present their concerns.

4. Changes or modifications accepted by the NCP/SL Committeewill be integrated into the list that is re-published on an annual basis.

STAFFING:

Governance and Scientific Affairs and Research provide staff support to NCP/SL Committee and for Research Committee functions.

Attachments

1. Letter template for proposing a **New Term for Nutrition Diagnostic Terminology**
2. Letter template for proposing **Modifications to Nutrition Diagnostic Terminology**
3. Template for **Reference Sheet** to **support additions/modifications to Nutrition Diagnostic Terminology**
4. Completed **Reference Sheet Example (Case with PES statement not included)**

SUBJECT: NUTRITION CONTROLLED VOCABULARY/TERMINOLOGY MAINTENANCE/REVIEW

Attachment 1: Letter Template for Proposing a New Term for Nutrition Diagnostic Terminology

Date: ___________

To: NCP/SL Committee
Scientific Affairs and Research
American Dietetic Association
120 South Riverside Plaza, Suite 2000
Chicago, IL 60606-6995
emyers@eatright.org; cchanner@eatright.org

Subject: Proposed Addition to Nutrition Diagnostic Terminology

(I/We) would like to propose a new term, ____________________(Proposed term to add to the Nutrition Diagnostic Terminology list). The reason I/we believe that this term should be added is as follows (insert concise rationale for change and may include brief example of when the situation arose that the current term was inadequately defined):

1. (Insert first statement of rationale.)
2. (Insert second statement of rationale, if applicable.)
3. (Insert example of situation where this modification was needed.)

Other terms that are similar and explanations of why they do not exactly match our new proposed term are as follows:

1. (Insert number and name.) – (Insert 2-3 sentences to illustrate why the existing term does not meet your need.)
2. (Insert number and name.) – (Insert 2-3 sentences to illustrate why the existing term does not meet your need.)
3. (Add as many as applicable.)

Attached is the a reference sheet that includes the label, description, proposed domain and category, examples of etiologies and signs and symptoms and a case that illustrates when this term would be used and the corresponding PES statement that would be used in medical record documentation.

The point of contact for this proposal is ___________________________________ (insert name), who can be reached at ______(best contact telephone number) and ______(e-mail address).

Thank you for considering our request.

Signature block
(Organizational unit if applicable)

Attachments: (1) Completed Reference Sheet Template (Case and PES statement example not included)

SUBJECT: NUTRITION CONTROLLED VOCABULARY/TERMINOLOGY MAINTENANCE/REVIEW

Attachment 2: Letter Template for Proposing Modifications to Nutrition Diagnostic Terminology

Date: ____________________

To: NCP/SL Committee
Scientific Affairs and Research
American Dietetic Association
120 South Riverside Plaza, Suite 2000
Chicago, IL 60606-6995
emyers@eatright.org; cchanner@eatright.org

Subject: Proposed Modification to Existing Nutrition Diagnostic Terminology

(I/We) would like to propose a modification or the term, ____________________(insert Number and Name from current Nutrition Diagnostic Terminology list). The reason I/we believe that this term should be modified is as follows (insert concise rationale for change and may include brief example of when the situation arose that the current term was inadequately defined):

1. (Insert first statement of rationale.)
2. (Insert second statement of rationale, if applicable.)
3. (Insert example of situation where this modification was needed.)

Attached is the revised reference sheet which shows the changes highlighted or bolded for your consideration.

The point of contact for this proposal is ___________________________________ (insert name), who can be reached at ______(best contact telephone number) and _______(e-mail address).

Thank you for considering our request.

Signature block
(Organizational unit if applicable)

Attachments: (1) Completed Reference Sheet Template

SUBJECT: NUTRITION CONTROLLED VOCABULARY/TERMINOLOGY MAINTENANCE/REVIEW

Attachment 3: Template for Reference Sheet for New Term or Proposing Modifications

[Select DOMAIN: CLINICAL/FUNCTIONAL or BEHAVIORAL/ENVIRONMENTAL]

[Select Category, e.g., Functional Balance]

Nutrition Diagnostic Label [Leave number blank, if new term.]

[Insert a 1-4 word label.]

Definition of Nutrition Diagnostic Label
[Insert 1 sentence or bullet that describes the intent of the new or modified label.]

Etiology *(Cause/Contributing Risk Factors)*
Factors gathered during the nutrition assessment process that contribute to the existence of or the maintenance of pathophysiological, psychosocial, situational, developmental, cultural, and/or environmental problems:

- **[Insert common etiologies for Nutrition Diagnostic Label]**

Signs/Symptoms (***Defining Characteristics***) A typical cluster of subjective and objective signs and symptoms gathered during the nutrition assessment process that provide evidence that a problem exists; quantify the problem and describe its severity.

Nutrition Assessment Category	Potential Indicators of this Nutrition Diagnosis (one or more must be present)
Biochemical Data	• [Insert as appropriate.]
Anthropometric Measurements	• [Insert as appropriate.]
Physical Exam Findings	• [Insert as appropriate.]
Food/Nutrition History	• [Insert as appropriate.]
Client History	• [Insert as appropriate.]

SUBJECT: NUTRITION CONTROLLED VOCABULARY/TERMINOLOGY MAINTENANCE/REVIEW

Attachment 4: Template for Completed Reference Sheet

DOMAIN: CLINICAL/FUNCTIONAL

Category: Functional Balance

Nutrition Diagnostic Label (NC-1.1.)

Swallowing difficulty.

Definition of Nutrition Diagnostic Label

Impaired movement of food and liquid from the mouth to the stomach.

Etiology *(Cause/Contributing Risk Factors)*

Factors gathered during the nutrition assessment process that contribute to the existence of or the maintenance of pathophysiological, psychosocial, situational, developmental, cultural, and/or environmental problems:

- Mechanical causes such as inflammation; surgery; stricture; or oral, pharyngeal and esophageal tumors
- Motor causes, e.g., neurological or muscular disorders such as cerebral palsy, stroke, multiple sclerosis, scleroderma, or prematurity

Signs/Symptoms (***Defining Characteristics***) A typical cluster of subjective and objective signs and symptoms gathered during the nutrition assessment process that provide evidence that a problem exists; quantify the problem and describe its severity.

Nutrition Assessment Category	Potential Indicators of this Nutrition Diagnosis (one or more must be present)
Biochemical Data	
Anthropometric Measurements	
Physical Exam Findings	• Evidence of dehydration, e.g., dry mucous membranes, poor skin turgor
Food/Nutrition History	Observations or reports of: • Coughing, choking, prolonged chewing, pouching of food, regurgitation, facial expression changes during eating, prolonged feeding time, drooling, noisy wet upper airway sounds, feeling of fo od getting stuck, pain while swallowing • Decreased food intake • Avoidance of foods • Mealtime resistance
Client History	• Conditions associated with a diagnosis or treatment of dysphagia, achalasia • Radiological findings, e.g., abnormal swallowing studies • Repeated upper respiratory infections and/or pneumonia

2003-2005 Standardized Language Task Force and Terminology Expert Reviewers

Standardized Language Task Force

Chair
Sylvia Escott-Stump, MA, RD, LDN
Dietetic Programs Director
East Carolina University
155 Rivers Building, Dept. NUHM
Greenville, NC 27858
Task Force Member 2003-2005

Peter Beyer, MS, RD, LD
Associate Professor
University of Kansas Medical Center
7315 Rosewood Drive
Prairie Village, KS 66208-2458
Task Force Member 2003-2005

Christina Biesemeier MS, RD, LDN, FADA
313 Logans Circle
Franklin TN 37067-1363
Task Force Member 2003-2005

Pam Charney, MS, RD, CNSD
2460 64th Ave SE
Mercer Island, WA 98040
Task Force Member 2003-2005

Marion Franz, MS, RD, CDE
6635 Limerick Dr.
Minneapolis, MN 55439-1260
Task Force Member 2003-2005

Karen Lacey, MS, RD, CD
500 Saint Mary's Blvd
Green Bay, WI 54301-2610
Task Force Member 2003-2005

Kathleen Niedert, MBA, RD, LD, FADA
PO Box 843
110 Ardis Street
Hudson, IA 50643-0843
Task Force Member 2003-2005

Mary Jane Oakland, PhD, RD, LD, FADA
1612 Truman Drive
Ames, IA 50010-4344
Task Force Member 2003-2005

Patricia Splett, PhD, MPH, RD
Splett & Associates
3219 Midland Avenue
St. Paul, MN 55110
Task Force Member 2003-2005

Frances Tyus, MS, RD, LD
19412 Mayfair Ln
Cleveland, OH 44128-2727
Task Force Member 2003-2005

Naomi Trostler, PhD, RD
Institute of Biochemistry, Food Science, and Nutrition
Faculty of Agriculture, Food and Environmental Quality Sciences
The Hebrew University of Jerusalem
PO Box 12
Rehovot 76100, Israel
Task Force Member 2004-2005

Robin Leonhardt, RD
1905 North 24th Street
Sheboygan, WI 53081-2124
Attended Face to Face Meeting in Summer 2003

Staff Liaisons
Esther Myers, PhD, RD, FADA
Director of Scientific Affairs and Research
ADA Headquarters
120 South Riverside Plaza, Suite 2000
Chicago, IL 60606-6995
Work (312) 899-4860
Fax (312) 899-4757
E-mail: emyers@eatright.org

Ellen Pritchett, RD, CPHQ
Director, Quality and Outcomes
ADA Headquarters
120 South Riverside Plaza, Suite 2000
Chicago, IL 60606-6995
Work (312) 899-4823
Fax (312) 899-4757
E-mail: epritchett@eatright.org
Staff Liaison 2003-2005

Lt Col Vivian Hutson, MA, MHA, RD, LD, Fellow,
American College of Healthcare Executives
Staff Liaison 2003-2004

2003-2005 Standardized Language Task Force and Terminology Expert Reviewers

Consultants

Donna G. Pertel, MEd, RD
5 Bonny Lane
Clinton, CT 06413

Patricia Splett, PhD, MPH, RD
Splett & Associates
3219 Midland Avenue
St. Paul, MN 55110

Melinda L. Jenkins, Ph.D., FNP
Assistant Professor of Clinical Nursing
Columbia University School of Nursing
630 W. 168 St., mail code 6
New York, NY 10032

Annalynn Skipper, MS, RD, FADA
P.O. Box 45
Oak Park, IL 60303

Expert Reviewers
Nutrition Diagnosis Labels

Nutrition Diagnostic Label	Dx Label #	Reviewers
CLINICAL DOMAIN – Functional Balance		
Swallowing difficulty	NC-1.1	Moshe Shike, MD (Memorial Sloan Kettering)
Chewing (masticatory) difficulty	NC-1.2	Helen Smiciklas-Wright, PhD, RD (Penn State) Riva Touger-Decker, PhD, RD (UMDNJ)
Breastfeeding difficulty	NC-1.3	Maureen A. Murtaugh, PhD, RD (University of Utah)
Altered GI function	NC-1.4	Larry Cheskin, MD (Johns Hopkins)
CLINICAL DOMAIN – Biochemical Balance		
Impaired nutrient utilization	NC-2.1	Laura Matarese, MS, RD, CNSD (Cleveland Clinic)
Altered nutrition-related laboratory values	NC-2.2	Denise Baird Schwartz, MS, RD, CNSD (Clinical practice)
Food-medication interaction	NC-2.3	Andrea Hutchins, PhD, RD (Arizona State University East, Mesa, AZ)
CLINICAL DOMAIN – Weight Balance		
Underweight	NC-3.1	Bonnie Spear, PhD, RD (University of Alabama, Birmingham)
Involuntary weight loss	NC-3.2	Jody Vogelzang, MS, RD, LD, CD, FADA (Texas Women's University)
Overweight/obesity	NC-3.3	Rebecca Mullis, PhD, RD (Georgia)
Involuntary weight gain	NC-3.4	Celia Hayes, MS, RD (HRSA)
BEHAVIORAL-ENVIRONMENTAL DOMAIN – Knowledge and Beliefs		
Food- and nutrition-related knowledge deficit	NB-1.1	Penny Kris-Etherton, PhD, RD (Penn State)
Harmful beliefs/attitudes about food, nutrition, and nutrition-related topics	NB-1.2	Keith-Thomas Ayoob, PhD, RD (Albert Einstein)
Not ready for diet/lifestyle change	NB-1.3	Geoffrey Greene, PhD, RD (University of Rhode Island)
Self-monitoring deficit	NB-1.4	Linda Delahanty, MS, RD (Harvard)
Disordered eating pattern	NB-1.5	Eileen Stellefson Myers, PhD, RD (Private practice) Leah Graves, MS, RD (Saint Francis Hospital, Tulsa, OK)
Limited adherence to nutrition-related recommendations	NB-1.6	Ellen Parham, PhD, RD (Northern IL)
Undesirable food choices	NB-1.7	Kathy Cobb, MS, RD (Centers for Disease Control)
BEHAVIORAL-ENVIRONMENTAL DOMAIN – Physical Activity Balance and Function		
Physical inactivity	NB-2.1	Melinda Manore, PhD, RD (Oregon State)
Excessive exercise	NB-2.2	Katherine Beals, PhD, RD (Industry, formerly Ball State)
Inability to manage self-care	NB-2.3	Emily Gier, MS, RD (Cornell)
Impaired ability to prepare foods/meals	NB-2.4	Marla Reicks, PhD, RD (U of MN)
Poor nutrition quality of life	NB-2.5	Elvira Johnson, MS, RD (Private practice)
Self-feeding difficulty	NB-2.6	Mary Cluskey, PhD, RD (Oregon State)
BEHAVIORAL-ENVIRONMENTAL DOMAIN – Food Safety and Access		
Intake of unsafe food	NB-3.1	Johanna Dwyer, DSc, RD (Tufts)
Limited access to food	NB-3.2	Sondra King, PhD, RD (Northern Illinois University)
INTAKE DOMAIN – Caloric Energy Balance		
Hypermetabolism	NI-1.1	Jonathan Waitman, MD for Louis Arrone, MD

2003-2005 Standardized Language Task Force and Terminology Expert Reviewers

		(Cornell)
Increased energy expenditure (when part of hypermetabolism)	NI-1.2	Jonathan Waitman, MD for Louis Arrone, MD (Cornell)
Hypometabolism	NI-1.3	Edith Lerner, PhD (Case Western Reserve University)
Inadequate energy intake	NI-1.4	Joel Mason, MD (Tufts)
Excessive energy intake	NI-1.5	Jim Hill, MD (University of Colorado)
INTAKE DOMAIN – Oral or Nutrition Support Intake		
Inadequate oral food/beverage intake	NI-2.1	Anne Voss, PhD, RD (Ross Labs)
Excessive oral food/beverage intake	NI-2.2	Jessica Krenkel, MS, RD (University of Nevada)
Inadequate intake from enteral/parenteral nutrition	NI-2.3	Kenneth Kudsk, MD (University of Wisconsin)
Excessive intake from enteral/parenteral nutrition	NI-2.4	Annalynn Skipper, MS, RD (University of Nebraska Lincoln)
Inappropriate infusion of enteral/parenteral nutrition	NI-2.5	Annalynn Skipper, MS, RD (University of Nebraska-Lincoln)
INTAKE DOMAIN – Fluid Intake Balance		
Inadequate fluid intake	NI-3.1	Ann Grandjean, EdD, RD (International Center for Sports Nutrition)
Excessive fluid intake	NI-3.2	Joel Kopple, MD (UCLA)
INTAKE DOMAIN – Bioactive Substances Intake Balance		
Inadequate bioactive substance intake	NI-4.1	Johanna Lappe, PhD, RN (Creighton)
Excess bioactive substance	NI-4.2	Elizabeth Jeffery, PhD (Univ. of IL, Champaign)
Excessive alcohol intake	NI-4.3	Janice Harris, PhD, RD (University of Kansas)
INTAKE DOMAIN – Nutrient Intake Balance		
Increased nutrient needs (specify)	NI-5.1	Carol Braunschweig, PhD, RD (University of Illinois, Chicago)
Evident protein-energy malnutrition	NI-5.2	Charlette R. Gallagher Allred, PhD, RD (Retired-Ross Labs)
Inadequate protein energy intake	NI-5.3	Trisha Fuhrman, MS, RD, FADA, CNSD (Coram, Inc.)
Decreased nutrient needs (specify)	NI-5.4	Jeannmarie Beiseigel, PhD, RD (USDA)
Imbalance of nutrients	NI-5.5	Molly Kretsch, PhD, RD (USDA)
INTAKE DOMAIN – Nutrient Balance – Fat and Cholesterol Balance		
Inadequate fat intake	NI-51.1	Alice Lichtenstein, DSc (Tufts)
Excessive fat intake	NI-51.2	Wendy Mueller Cunnigham, PhD, RD (Cal State)
Inappropriate intake of food fats	NI-51.3	Nancy Lewis, PhD, RD (University of Nebraska-Lincoln)
INTAKE DOMAIN – Nutrient Balance – Protein Balance		
Inadequate protein intake	NI-52.1	Don Layman, PhD (University of Illinois-Champaign)
Excessive or unbalanced protein intake	NI-52.2	Linda A. Vaughan, PhD, RD (Arizona State)
Inappropriate intake of amino acids	NI-52.3	Allison Yates, PhD, RD (Industry, formerly Director of the IOM Food and Nutrition Board)
INTAKE DOMAIN – Nutrient Balance – Carbohydrate Balance		
Inadequate carbohydrate intake	NI-53.1	Robert Wolfe, PhD (University of Texas Medical Branch)
Excessive carbohydrate intake	NI-53.2	Anne Daly, MS, RD
Inappropriate intake of types of carbohydrate	NI-53.3	Lyn Wheeler, MS, RD, CD, FADA, CDE (Indiana University School of Medicine)
Inconsistent intake of carbohydrate	NI-53.4	Maggie Powers, MS, RD, CDE (International Diabetes Center)
Inadequate fiber intake	NI-53.5	Joanne Slavin, PhD, RD (University of Minnesota)
Excess fiber intake	NI-53.6	Judith Marlett, PhD, RD (University of Wisconsin)
INTAKE DOMAIN – Nutrient Balance – Vitamin Balance		
Inadequate vitamin intake (specify)	NI-54.1	Laurie A. Kruzich, MS, RD (Iowa State) Kristina Penniston, PhD, RD (University of Wisconsin)

Excess vitamin intake (specify)	NI-54.2	Kristina Penniston, PhD, RD (University of Wisconsin)
INTAKE DOMAIN – Nutrient Balance – Mineral Balance		
Inadequate mineral intake (specify)	NI-55.1	Bob Heaney, MD (Creighton)
Excessive mineral intake (specify)	NI-55.2	Joan Fischer, PhD, RD (University of Georgia)

Implementing Nutrition Diagnosis, Step Two in the Nutrition Care Process and Model: Challenges and Lessons Learned in Two Health Care Facilities

Jennifer Mathieu; Mandy Foust, RD; Patricia Ouellette, RD

In adherence to the American Dietetic Association's (ADA) Strategic Plan goal of establishing and implementing a standardized Nutrition Care Process (NCP) in the hopes of "increasing demand and utilization of services provided by members" (1), dietetics professionals in two health care facilities established an NCP pilot program in 2005, in collaboration with ADA. The pilot sites were the Virginia Hospital Center in Arlington and the Veterans Affairs Medical Center in San Diego, CA.

This article gives a background on the NCP and model, the standardized language used in the nutrition diagnosis step, medical record documentation, and an explanation of how the two sites came to participate in the pilot program. It also provides a timeline for each site's implementation of the NCP, including challenges faced and lessons learned. Similarities and differences in approaches will also be discussed. Managers from both facilities will offer advice to facilities who are contemplating implementation of the NCP and nutrition diagnoses in the future.

BACKGROUND

ADA developed a four-step NCP and Model that appeared in the August 2003 issue of the *Journal*. The NCP consists of four "distinct but interrelated and connected steps"—Nutrition Assessment, Nutrition Diagnosis, Nutrition Intervention, and Nutrition Monitoring and Evaluation (2). The NCP and Model were developed by the Quality Management Committee Work Group with input from the House of Delegates.

This new model calls for dietetics professionals to incorporate a new step—making a nutrition diagnosis—which involves working with defined terminology. It also asks dietetics professionals to chart their diagnosis in the form of a statement that establishes the patient's problem (diagnostic label), etiology (cause/contributing risk factors), and signs and symptoms (defining characteristics). This is known as a PESS statement, and makes up the heart of the NCP's second step—nutrition diagnosis.

"The second step is the culture shift," says Susan Ramsey, MS, RD, CDE, LDN, senior manager of medical nutrition services for Sodexho who also serves on ADA's Research Committee. "The second step forces us to make a one-line statement. It brings the whole assessment into one clear vision."

According to the article by Lacey and Pritchett, using the new model provides many benefits. The model defines a common language that allows nutrition practice to be more measurable, creates a format that enables the process to generate quantitative and qualitative data that can then be analyzed and interpreted, serves as the structure to validate nutrition care, and shows how the care that was provided does what it intends to do (2). It also gives the profession a greater sense of autonomy, says Ramsey. "It's given us responsibility for our work instead of looking for permission from others."

The nutrition diagnostic labels and reference sheets were developed by the Standardized Language Task Force, chaired by Sylvia Escott-Stump, MA, RD, LDN. It is from this list that dietetics professionals utilizing the NCP list the P (problem) part of their PESS statement. According to Escott-Stump, this Standardized Language will help bring dietetics professionals a new focus and the ability to target their interventions into more effective results that will match the patient nutrition diagnosis (problem).

It is Escott-Stump's belief that documenting nutrition diagnoses, interventions, and outcomes will allow for dietetics professionals to better track diagnoses over several clients, allowing the profession to be more likely to track the types of nutrition diagnoses that clients have, and be able to state that the profession affects certain types of acute and chronic diseases more than others.

"For example, now we believe that our impact on cardiovascular, endocrine, and renal diseases is strong, but we may find that our professionals impact gastrointestinal disorders the most," says Escott-Stump. "By having standardized language, we will be able to validate or correct our suspicions."

This pilot implementation of the nutrition care model also tested a new method of charting that differs from the traditional Subjective Objective Assessment Plan format (SOAP). The new ADI template stands for Assessment, Diagnosis, and Intervention (including Monitoring and Evaluation).

According to Dr Esther Myers,

***J. Mathieu** is xxx, Houston, TX. **M. Foust** is xxx. **P. Ouellette** is xxx.*

Address correspondence to: Jennifer Mathieu, 5639 Berry Creek Dr, Houston, TX 77017. E-mail: jenmathieu27@yahoo.com
0002-8223/05/xx0x-0000$30.00/0
doi: 10.1016/j.jada.2005.07.015

PhD, RD, FADA, ADA's Research and Scientific Affairs director, ADA plans to expand these two pilot tests through the Peer Network for Nutrition Diagnosis in the next 2 years. This group of dietetics professionals will receive additional training and networking opportunities to assist them as they implement this new model within their facility and then share their knowledge with other dietetics professionals in their geographical region.

Their experience will be used to determine what additional implementation tools are needed. In addition, a formal research project will be conducted through the Dietetics Practice Based Research Network in early 2006.

IMPLEMENTATION OF THE PROGRAM

Virginia Hospital Center

Mandy Foust, RD and Clinical Nutrition Manager of the Virginia Hospital Center, is contracted through Sodexho to oversee patient services at the 400-bed facility. In December 2004, Foust, who had learned about PESS statements while in school, decided to have her college dietetic intern Anne Avery research current changes and updates in charting for dietetics professionals.

Avery spoke with Dr Myers and discussed the possibility of the Virginia Hospital Center serving as a pilot site for the new model. Foust was excited about the idea for several reasons. "To me, the nutrition care model is a clinically based, concise way of charting that sets goals and is more standardized with other disciplines," she says. Until the implementation of the pilot project, the RDs on staff at the Virginia Hospital Center used the SOAP format of charting.

A conference call took place between Foust, Dr Myers, Avery, and Avery's internship director at Virginia Tech. Foust selected one of her five inpatient registered dietitians (RDs) to serve as the first RD to use the new method. It was decided Avery would present an in-service on the nutrition care model to the dietetics professionals on staff. This in-service provided the RDs with introductory information, the four steps of the NCP, PESS statements, diagnostic labeling, and why the changes would be beneficial.

Foust says there were concerns from her staff about the new method. These included that the new ADI charting format would not allow them to be thorough enough and that it seemed "too cookie cutter." Staff also expressed concern that it would be difficult to sum up two or more serious problems in one PESS statement. They also worried that physicians would be wary of the term "nutrition diagnosis."

Over several days in mid-December, Foust arranged meetings with several hospital administrators, including the vice president of the hospital, the chief nursing officer, the medical staff president, and the chief of the nutrition committee to get their feedback on the pilot project. She also kept her supervisor at Sodexho abreast of the situation. "Because I am a contractor, I want to make sure I'm covering my bases," says Foust. She says the Virginia Hospital Center is "very interdisciplinary" and that she wanted there to be an awareness of the upcoming changes.

Administrators initially had questions about how the new method would benefit patients, but Foust says after she met with them and presented them with information on the nutrition care model, they were receptive to the changes. The physician who served as chief of the hospital's nutrition committee had concerns about the idea of a nutrition diagnosis. Foust says she reassured him that the new method did not ask RDs to make a medical diagnosis or interfere with a physician's orders.

After the nutrition committee approved the project in early January 2005, Foust was asked to inform several other hospital staff members about the new format, including the chief of surgery and the chief of surgical education. Because the first RD to participate in the pilot project worked in the intensive care unit (ICU), Foust was also asked to notify the medical director of the ICU, two ICU nurse educators, and the ICU patient care director via formal letters. Responses to these letters encouraged Foust to seek approval for the project from the hospital's patient-monitoring committee.

During the end of January while waiting for a response from the patient-monitoring committee, Foust met for about an hour each week with the RD who would be the first to use the new method. The RD used actual patients from her daily census to begin practicing PESS statements and ADI charting. Foust shared the results with Dr Myers and the Standardized Language Task Force often. Through early to mid-February the RD submitted her notes in both the SOAP format and the new format as a way of practicing the new method.

At the end of January, the patient-monitoring committee gave the project its approval. Before implementation officially occurred, Foust requested permission and modified the Hakel-Smith Coding Instrument as an auditing tool to evaluate the charts. She also developed a questionnaire for allied health professionals to give feedback on the new system of charting.

On February 16, 2005, the ICU RD, Korinne Umbaugh, officially began submitting all of her notes using the ADI template. Foust audited two to three charts each day. In late February, a second RD began using the new method of charting. On March 28, a third RD began the process. By the middle of April, all five RDs were using the ADI template, with the fifth RD beginning the process on the second week of the month.

Throughout the entire transition Foust met formally and informally with staff RDs both individually and in groups. Foust says at least 20 minutes of each weekly hour-long staff meeting continues to be spent discussing the new method of charting and reviewing PESS statements. At this time Foust is editing about 10% of the charts.

Unfortunately, Foust did not receive as many completed questionnaires as she hoped for from allied health professionals. However, her initial chart audits showed that by the end of April the staff had become much more comfortable with the process. Audits revealed notes that steadily became more direct and concise, as well as more outcome-oriented. Extraneous information was not included as often.

Veterans Affairs Medical Center, San Diego

Patricia Ouellette, RD, is the deputy director of nutrition and food services for the Veterans Affairs Medical Center in San Diego, CA. The Medical Center is a 238-bed facility. There are three RDs who focus on the inpatient areas of the facility.

In January 2004, the facility's director of nutrition and food service, Ginger Hughes, MS, RD, distributed the August 2003 article by Karen Lacey, MS, RD and Ellen Pritchett, RD, about the NCP that appeared in the *Journal*. The staff was advised to read the article and become familiar with it. In the fall of 2004, internship program director Tere Bush-Zurn and outpatient dietitian Teresa Hilleary received a scholarship to attend the Nutrition Diagnosis Roundtable for Educators workshop at the ADA's 2004 Food and Nutrition Conference and Exhibition. Bush-Zurn and Hilleary relayed what they learned with the rest of their staff when they returned to California.

In November 2004, a staff meeting is held to discuss questions and concerns surrounding the NCP and PESS statements. The staff agreed to start using the PESS statements as soon as possible. After a December 2004 workshop presented by a visiting Lacey, the staff agreed that they wanted to work toward transitioning to the nutrition care model and would serve as a pilot site.

"It evolved after a year of looking at the process and after a lot of discussions with the staff," says Ouellette. "We are a teaching institution and we wanted to challenge ourselves in terms of our practice. We also have a dietetic internship program and feel responsible for providing the interns with the most progressive concepts in our field of practice."

As with the Virginia Hospital Center RDs, the RDs at the VA had been using the SOAP format for many years and they had similar concerns over whether the new method would be deemed thorough enough. They were also concerned that one PESS statement would not be enough if the patient had several complicated problems.

Based on staff consensus, in February 2005 the staff started devoting time at the weekly staff meeting to discussing issues related to the new method. The staff practiced writing PESS statements and shared the results with each other during this time. They also discussed questions and concerns related to the new method.

At the same time, several staff members, including the staff's performance improvement/information technology dietitian, worked separately to develop a point-and-click computer version of the inpatient initial nutrition assessment ADI template that could be used by the inpatient RDs on staff when writing their notes.

During the last week in March, the inpatient RDs spent 1 week writing their notes using both the old SOAP method and the new template. On April 4, the staff officially implemented the new version of charting for the inpatient initial nutrition assessments and stopped using the SOAP method completely. For the first month after the official implementation, Ouellette checked every inpatient initial nutrition assessment chart note and provided weekly feedback to the staff.

In May, the auditing components were incorporated into the NFS Periodic Performance Review plan implemented as part of the Joint Commission on Accreditation of Healthcare Organizations' continuous readiness philosophy. Although not required, they believed this was a good way to continue to audit and document the process.

Ouellette continued to meet with RDs individually as problems and questions developed about the change. Her initial audits revealed that the majority of the staff uses the same five to six diagnostic labels. She also assessed that after 2 weeks of using the new ADI template exclusively, PESS statements markedly improved and chart notes became more focused and concise. After 3 weeks the amount of time spent on the notes shortened, suggesting that the staff was becoming more comfortable with the process.

In regard to diagnostic labels, Ouellette's staff began the practice of utilizing two diagnostic labels and combining them into one PESS statement if the two conditions were closely related (eg, difficulty swallowing and chewing difficulty).

The monitoring component of the process still needs to be observed carefully, as many of Ouellette's staff members are not yet in the habit of stating which specific laboratory tests need to be performed.

SIMILARITIES AND DIFFERENCES

The biggest difference between the two sites was the time spent seeking approval for the project before proceeding. As a contractor, Foust believed she needed to secure approval from several different administrators before beginning implementation. Ouellette's approval process occurred much more informally. Ouellette says this is because the VA allows flexibility in how Nutrition and Food Services' processes are carried out.

Another difference centered on the way staff RDs began participating in the implementation. Ouellette's staff discussed the process for about a year before they all began the new method of charting at the same time. Ouellette and her staff wanted to work with only one inpatient charting template at a time, and this allowed them to do so. Also, Ouellette believed that if the SOAP method template was available, RDs might be tempted to go back to the old format that they felt most comfortable using.

After the staff in-service, Foust started one of her RDs on the new method and others followed over a period of months. As the implementation was occurring, the staff had several meetings to discuss the new changes. Foust believed this gradual method of implementation allowed time for RDs who were having trouble with the new method to learn from RDs who were actively working with it.

The similarities between both sites included the increased amount of administrative time spent on the change (especially at the manager level) as well as the decision to focus the change to inpatient areas only. Foust and Ouellette both said this decision was made because inpatient cases tend to be more complex, and if these cases could be dealt with successfully it would be even easier to make the transition with outpatient cases. The sites shared another similarity in that the types of concerns held by the staffs were nearly identical, as were the challenges they faced and the lessons they learned.

CHALLENGES AND LESSONS LEARNED

According to Foust and Ouellette, the biggest challenge for both sites was assisting their RDs in completely changing the way they think about their chart notes. "It's a brand new language," says Foust. "My RDs are already seeing 14, 16 patients a day, and it's a long process when you're starting something new."

Both managers say their RDs had a hard time excluding extraneous language. In the SOAP format, for example, RDs were used to including information about everything from decades-old surgeries, the patient's general mood, and other aspects of the patient's condition that are not relevant to a nutrition diagnosis. With the nutrition care model, the charting must be much more exact. "This new method requires us to focus on establishing a nutrition label and forces us to restrict our charting to what is relevant to that nutritional diagnosis," says Ouellette.

Also challenging for the RDs was the creation of the PESS statements. "They initially roadblock with the PESS," says Foust. "It is a completely different way of formatting your thoughts. It's moving from a very conversational way of charting to a more clinical-sounding, concise note. This results in a struggle when first charting."

Staff members at both sites had concerns over what to do when there seemed to be two separate but equally important problems. After discussions with Dr Myers, it was decided that, on occasion, two PESS statements can be used.

Ouellette adds that another challenge comes from the fact that the nutrition care model means a different way of approaching formatting the chart note. "The chart note really has to be decided after determining the PESS statement," says Ouellette. "The statement can only be determined after a thorough nutritional assessment. The chart review and patient consultation method are the same, but the structuring of the chart note is quite different. We no longer do this in a linear fashion. We start from the middle with the PESS statement and complete both ends—assessment and goals—from there."

RDs also struggled with how to write PESS statements for patients that simply had no nutrition risk. Foust says she urged her staff to recognize that if they were experts in making a nutrition diagnosis, they could say that at certain times there is no nutrition diagnosis. Ouellette adds that it might be a good idea to create a category of "potential" diagnostic labels that could be used for patients who are basically stable with tube feedings or dialysis, but who still need to be monitored.

While the PESS statement proved to be the most difficult hurdle, RDs also had to learn to be more specific when it came time to express how they would monitor and evaluate their patients. It wasn't enough to write "monitor labs," says Foust. "You need to give specific labs and then follow with an explanation and expected outcomes."

For managers, keeping morale of staff up was a challenge. This was especially true for RDs who spoke of feeling stifled by the new method and who constantly feared they were making a mistake. Managers learned they needed to spend extra time encouraging their RDs and reminding them that they were working on a cutting-edge project.

"All of my RDs are competent and brilliant," says Foust. "Changing the way they chart and implementing new techniques can cause doubt. This can potentially alter their clinical self confidence, and you want to maintain a positive outlook to avoid this."

Both Foust and Ouellette say it was beneficial to work in groups on PESS statements and learn from each other, being sure to highlight well-written charts as well as the ones that that needed attention. Foust and Ouellette also learned that not every RD would learn at the same pace. While RDs who had been in the profession for a shorter amount of time were often able to grasp the concept faster, Ouellette adds that, in general, the RDs who had the easiest time were the ones with personality types that adjusted well to change, regardless of experience level.

ADVICE TO SITES READY FOR IMPLEMENTATION

Both Foust and Ouellette offer similar advice to sites seeking to implement the NCP and model. Both suggest an in-service for the staff and the distribution of materials well ahead of implementation. Ouellette also suggests providing training from a knowledgeable source, as was the case with Karen Lacey speaking to her staff using ADA slides describing the NCP.

Both managers suggest setting aside a generous portion of the weekly staff meeting time to discuss the model, review PESS statements, answer questions, and motivate the staff with positive feedback.

While Foust and Ouellette had different experiences in terms of seeking approval from the administration to implement the program, both suggest allowing time to meet with the necessary people in the facility, as the approval needed will differ from facility to facility.

Most of all, Ouellette and Foust suggest that future managers and staffs remind themselves that transitioning to the nutrition care model is a beneficial but time-consuming process that requires patience. Both say they have seen marked improvements among their staff over time, and many of the initial challenges have been overcome with patience and practice.

"You're changing the way you're thinking, you're changing the way you're charting, it's a huge change," says Ouellette. "There are no shortcuts you can take. But my staff is excited about being on the forefront. It's certainly a worthwhile thing."

Adds Foust, "This continues to be an excellent groundbreaking experience."

The authors would like to acknowledge the contributions of the following people in the preparation of this article: Susan Ramsey, MS, RD, CDE, LDN, senior manager of medical nutrition services for Sodexho who also serves on ADA's Research Committee; Sylvia Escott-Stump MA, RD, LDN, Standardized Language Task Force Chair; and Esther Myers, PhD, RD, FADA, ADA's Research and Scientific Affairs director.

References

1. American Dietetic Association Strategic Plan. Available at: http://www.eatright.org (member-only section). Accessed April 17, 2005.
2. Lacey K, Pritchett E. Nutrition Care Process and Model: ADA adopts road map to quality care and outcomes management. *J Am Diet Assoc.* 2003;103:1061-1072.

TIMELINES OF IMPLEMENTATION

Virginia Hospital Center

December 2004

- Idea of participating in pilot project presented to facility.
- Staff in-service held to educate staff about the NCP, ADI charting, and PESS statements.
- Meetings between clinical nutrition manager and hospital administrators to discuss the NCP and seek approval for participation in the pilot project.

January 2005

- Hospital nutrition committee approves the pilot project.
- Other hospital administrators, including those on the unit where the first RD to participate in the project works, are informed of the pilot project.
- The hospital's patient-monitoring committee approves the pilot project.
- Throughout the month of January, the first RD to take part in the project meets regularly with clinical nutrition manager to practice ADI charting and PESS statements.
- Clinical nutrition manager obtains permission and modifies the Hakel-Smith Coding Instrument as a way of auditing charts.

February 2005

- From early to mid-February, the first RD to participate in the project charts using both the ADI and SOAP formats before formally transitioning to the ADI method alone on February 16.
- In late February, a second RD begins to exclusively use the ADI method of charting.

March 2005

- By the end of March, a third RD has transitioned to the ADI method of charting.
- Throughout the entire process, the clinical nutrition manager meets formally and informally with RDs both individually and in groups to discuss concerns and monitor progress.
- Throughout the process, at least 20 minutes of each weekly staff meeting are devoted to reviewing the ADI method of charting, PESS statements, questions, and concerns.

April 2005

- By the start of April, a fourth RD is exclusively using the ADI method of charting, with the fifth and final RD making the transition by mid-April.
- The clinical nutrition manager audits 10% of charts.

Veterans Affairs Medical Center, San Diego

January 2004

- Director of nutrition and food services distributes journal articles about the NCP to staff.

October 2004

- Two staff members attend the Nutrition Diagnosis Roundtable for Educators workshop at ADA's Food and Nutrition Conference and Exhibition and share what they learn with the rest of the staff upon their return.

November 2004

- A staff meeting is held to discuss questions and concerns surrounding the NCP and PESS statements.

December 2004

- ADA's Karen Lacey, Chair of ADA's Quality Management Working Group on the NCP, provides the staff with a workshop on the NCP.

February 2005

- The staff begins to devote time during each weekly staff meeting to practice using the new method and to share PESS statements.
- Several staff members, including the staff's performance improvement/information technology dietitian, develop a point-and-click computer version of the ADI template for the staff to use.

March 2005

- Toward the end of March, the staff spends 1 week using both the SOAP format and the new ADI template to chart notes.

April 2005

- On April 4, the staff officially implements the new method of charting exclusively.
- The deputy director of nutrition and food service checks each inpatient initial nutrition assessment chart note and provides feedback to individuals.

May 2005

- Ongoing auditing was accomplished by incorporating the auditing elements into the periodic performance review plan implemented to ensure continuous readiness for the Joint Commission on Accreditation of Healthcare Organization's review.

NUTRITION CARE PROCESS AND MODEL WORK GROUP

Karen Lacey, MS, RD, Chair
Elvira Johnson, MS, RD
Kessey Kieselhorst, MPA, RD
Mary Jane Oakland, PhD, RD, FADA
Carlene Russell, RD, FADA
Patricia Splett, PhD, RD, FADA
Staff Liaisons:
Harold Holler, RD
Esther Myers, PhD, RD, FADA
Ellen Pritchett, RD
Karri Looby, MS, RD

The work group would like to extend a special thank you to Marion Hammond, MS, and Naomi Trostler, PhD, RD, for their assistance in development of the NCP and Model.

STANDARDIZED LANGUAGE TASK FORCE

Sylvia Escott-Stump, MA, RD, LDN, Chair
Peter Beyer, MS, RD, LD
Christina Biesemeier MS, RD, LDN, FADA
Pam Charney, MS, RD, CNSD
Marion Franz, MS, RD, CDE
Karen Lacey, MS, RD, CD
Carrie LePeyre, RD, LDN
Kathleen Niedert, MBA, RD, LD, FADA
Mary Jane Oakland, PhD, RD, LD, FADA
Patricia Splett, PhD, MPH, RD
Frances Tyus, MS, RD, LD

The task force would like to extend a special thank you to Naomi Trostler, PhD, RD, FADA.

FEEDBACK FORM

We welcome feedback on revisions to this reference for Nutrition Diagnosing. After evaluating each section, please indicate whether you would recommend that the section should be included in the next edition. Following this, please identify other questions that you would like answered in the next version. Finally, any additional materials you would find helpful is appreciated. Thank you for your time.

Should the following items should be included in the next version:	**Please Check (✓) YES**	**NO**
The Nutrition Care Process: Nutrition Care Process and Model Article		
Development of Standardized Language: American Dietetic Association's Standardized Language Model/Current Status		
Introduction to Nutrition Diagnoses/Problems		
Nutrition Diagnosis Reference Sheets: Single page list of Nutrition Diagnostic Terminology		
Nutrition Diagnosis Terms and Definitions: Table of Contents for next document		
Nutrition Diagnosis Reference Sheets (128 pages)		
Procedure for Nutrition Controlled Vocabulary/Terminology Maintenance/Review		
Camera Ready Pocket Guide		

What questions would you like answered in the 2007 version?

What additional materials would be helpful in the 2007 version?

Please remove this form from packet and mail to:
Scientific Affairs and Research
Nutrition Care Process /Standardized Language Committee
American dietetic Association
120 South Riverside Plaza, Suite 2000
Chicago, IL 60606-6995

You can also email this information to: cchanner@eatright.org

NUTRITION DIAGNOSTIC TERMINOLOGY

NUTRITION DIAGNOSTIC TERMINOLOGY

INTAKE — NI

Defined as "actual problems related to intake of energy, nutrients, fluids, bioactive substances through oral diet or nutrition support"

Caloric Energy Balance (1)

Defined as "actual or estimated changes in energy (kcal)"

- ❑ Hypermetabolism (Increased energy needs) — NI-1.1
- ❑ Increased energy expenditure — NI-1.2
- ❑ Hypometabolism (Decreased energy needs) — NI-1.3
- ❑ Inadequate energy intake — NI-1.4
- ❑ Excessive energy intake — NI-1.5

Oral or Nutrition Support Intake (2)

Defined as "actual or estimated food and beverage intake from oral diet or nutrition support" compared with patient goal"

- ❑ Inadequate oral food/beverage intake — NI-2.1
- ❑ Excessive oral food/beverage intake — NI-2.2
- ❑ Inadequate intake from enteral/parenteral nutrition infusion — NI-2.3
- ❑ Excessive intake from enteral/parenteral nutrition — NI-2.4
- ❑ Inappropriate infusion of enteral/parenteral nutrition (use with caution) — NI-2.5

Fluid Intake (3)

Defined as "actual or estimated fluid intake compared with patient goal"

- ❑ Inadequate fluid intake — NI-3.1
- ❑ Excessive fluid intake — NI-3.2

Bioactive Substances Intake (4)

Defined as "actual or observed intake of bioactive substances, including single or multiple functional food components, ingredients, dietary supplements, alcohol"

- ❑ Inadequate bioactive substance intake — NI-4.1
- ❑ Excessive bioactive substance intake — NI-4.2
- ❑ Excessive alcohol intake — NI-4.3

Nutrient Intake (5)

Defined as "actual or estimated intake of specific nutrient groups or single nutrients as compared with desired levels"

- ❑ Increased nutrient needs — NI-5.1
  (specify) ______________
- ❑ Evident protein-energy malnutrition — NI-5.2
- ❑ Inadequate protein-energy intake — NI-5.3
- ❑ Decreased nutrient needs — NI-5.4
  (specify) ______________
- ❑ Imbalance of nutrients — NI-5.5

Fat and Cholesterol (51)

- ❑ Inadequate fat intake — NI-51.1
- ❑ Excessive fat intake — NI-51.2
- ❑ Inappropriate intake of food fats — NI-51.3
  (specify) ______________

Protein (52)

- ❑ Inadequate protein intake — NI-52.1
- ❑ Excessive protein intake — NI-52.2
- ❑ Inappropriate intake of amino acids — NI-52.3
  (specify) ______________

Carbohydrate and Fiber (53)

- ❑ Inadequate carbohydrate intake — NI-53.1
- ❑ Excessive carbohydrate intake — NI-53.2
- ❑ Inappropriate intake of types of carbohydrate — NI-53.3
  (specify) ______________
- ❑ Inconsistent carbohydrate intake — NI-53.4
- ❑ Inadequate fiber intake — NI-53.5
- ❑ Excessive fiber intake — NI-53.6

NUTRITION DIAGNOSTIC TERMINOLOGY

NUTRITION DIAGNOSTIC TERMINOLOGY

Vitamin (54)

- ❑ Inadequate vitamin intake (specify) — NI-54.1
- ❑ Excessive vitamin intake (specify) — NI-54.2
  - ❑ A ❑ C
  - ❑ Thiamin ❑ D
  - ❑ Riboflavin ❑ E
  - ❑ Niacin ❑ K
  - ❑ Folate ❑ Other ______________

Mineral (55)

- ❑ Inadequate mineral intake (specify) — NI-55.1
  - ❑ Calcium ❑ Iron
  - ❑ Potassium ❑ Zinc
  - ❑ Other ______________
- ❑ Excessive mineral intake (specify) — NI-55.2
  - ❑ Calcium ❑ Iron
  - ❑ Potassium ❑ Zinc
  - ❑ Other ______________

CLINICAL — NC

Defined as "nutritional findings/problems identified as related to medical or physical conditions"

Functional (1)

Defined as "change in physical or mechanical functioning that interferes with or prevents desired nutritional consequences"

- ❑ Swallowing difficulty — NC-1.1
- ❑ Chewing (masticatory) difficulty — NC-1.2
- ❑ Breastfeeding difficulty — NC-1.3
- ❑ Altered GI function — NC-1.4

Biochemical (2)

Defined as "change in capacity to metabolize nutrients as a result of medications, surgery, or as indicated by altered lab values"

- ❑ Impaired nutrient utilization — NC-2.1
- ❑ Altered nutrition-related laboratory values — NC-2.2
  (specify) ______________
- ❑ Food-medication interaction — NC-2.3

Weight (3)

Defined as "chronic weight or changed weight status when compared with usual or desired body weight"

- ❑ Underweight — NC-3.1
- ❑ Involuntary weight loss — NC-3.2
- ❑ Overweight/obesity — NC-3.3
- ❑ Involuntary weight gain — NC-3.4

BEHAVIORAL-ENVIRONMENTAL — NB

Defined as "nutritional findings/problems identified as related to knowledge, attitudes/beliefs, physical environment, or food supply and safety"

Knowledge and Beliefs (1)

Defined as "actual knowledge and beliefs as reported, observed, or documented"

- ❑ Food, nutritition, and nutrition-related knowledge deficit — NB-1.1
- ❑ Harmful beliefs/attitudes about food or nutrition-related topics (use with caution) — NB-1.2
- ❑ Not ready for diet/lifestyle change — NB-1.3
- ❑ Self-monitoring deficit — NB-1.4
- ❑ Disordered eating pattern — NB-1.5
- ❑ Limited adherence to nutrition-related recommendations — NB-1.6
- ❑ Undesirable food choices — NB-1.7

Physical Activity and Function (2)

Defined as "actual physical activity, self-care, and quality of life problems as reported, observed, or documented"

- ❑ Physical inactivity — NB-2.1
- ❑ Excessive exercise — NB-2.2
- ❑ Inability or lack of desire to manage self-care — NB-2.3
- ❑ Impaired ability to prepare foods/meals — NB-2.4
- ❑ Poor nutrition quality of life — NB-2.5
- ❑ Self-feeding difficulty — NB-2.6

Food Safety and Access (3)

Defined as "actual problems with food access or food safety"

- ❑ Intake of unsafe food — NB-3.1
- ❑ Limited access to food — NB-3.2